Current Topics in Radiography
Number 1

CURRENT TOPICS IN RADIOGRAPHY

Editorial Board

Current Topics in Radiography Number 1

Edited by

Audrey Paterson FCR, MSc, TDCR, DMU
Head of Department of Radiography,
Canterbury Christ Church College,
Canterbury, Kent, UK

and

Richard Price FCR, MSc
Director of Studies,
Division of Clinical Sciences,
University of Hertfordshire,
Hatfield, Hertfordshire, UK

W.B. SAUNDERS COMPANY LTD
London · Philadelphia · Toronto
Sydney · Tokyo

W.B. Saunders Company Ltd   24–28 Oval Road
London NW1 7DX, England

The Curtis Center
Independence Square West
Philadelphia, PA 19106–3399, USA

55 Horner Avenue
Toronto, Ontario M8Z 4X6, Canada

Harcourt Brace
(Australia) Pty Ltd
30–52 Smidmore Street
Marrickville, NSW 2204, Australia

Harcourt Brace Japan Inc.
Ichibancho Central Building
22–1 Ichibancho
Chiyoda-ku, Tokyo 102, Japan

British Library Cataloguing in Publication Data is available

ISBN 0–7020–1971–2

This book is printed on acid-free paper

Typeset by Phoenix Photosetting, Chatham, Kent
Printed and bound in Great Britain by the University Press, Cambridge

Contents

Contributors

David Baker   Department of Radiology, Hastings and Rother NHS Trust, The Conquest Hospital, St Leonards-on-Sea, East Sussex TN27 7RD, UK.

Jane A. Bates   Ultrasound Department, St James' University Hospital, Leeds LS9 7TF, UK.

Keith E. Britton   Professor of Nuclear Medicine and Consultant Physician, St Bartholomew's Hospital, West Smithfield, London EC1A 7BE, UK.

Diane Carney   Radiology Services Manager, Royal Hampshire County Hospital, Romsey Road, Winchester, Hants SO22 5DG, UK.

Alexander J.M. Cavenagh   Gludy, Brecon, Powys LD3 9PE, UK.

Rose Marie Conlon   Ultrasound Department, St James' University Hospital, Leeds LS9 7TF, UK.

Olive M. Deaville   205 Weston Way, Baldock, Herts SG7 6JG, UK.

David Dewitt   Superintendent II Radiographer, Department of Radiography, Blackpool Victoria Hospital, Whinney Heys Road, Blackpool, Lancs, UK.

Anthony R. Divers   X-ray Department, St Albans & Hemel Hempstead NHS Trust, Hemel Hempstead General Hospital, Hillfield Road, Hemel Hempstead, Herts HP2 4AD, UK.

Stephen A. Evans   Director of Marketing, The Ipswich Hospital NHS Trust, Heath Road, Ipswich, Suffolk IP4 5PD, UK.

Maria Granowska   Senior Lecturer in Nuclear Medicine and Honorary Consultant, St Bartholomew's Hospital, West Smithfield, London EC1A 7BE, UK.

Anne Hemingway   Professor/Honorary Consultant, Department of Diagnostic Radiology, Hammersmith Hospital, Du Cane Road, London W12 0HS, UK.

John Lowe   The Clinical PET Centre, St Thomas' Hospital, Lambeth Palace Road, London SE1 7EH, UK.

Nuala Martin   Business Manager/District Radiographer, Department of Diagnostic Radiology, Hammersmith Hospital, Du Cane Road, London W12 0HS, UK.

Lyn McKay   The Maidstone Hospital, Hermitage Lane, Barming ME16 9QQ, UK.

Elizabeth J. McLean   Business Manager, University College London Hospitals Trust, Chenies Mews, 25 Grafton Way, London WC1E 6DB, UK.

Susan G. Moore   Clinical Superintendent, MRI Suite, Nuffield Orthopaedic Centre, Windmill Road, Headington, Oxford OX3 7LD, UK.

Lorraine Nuttall   Radiography Manager, X-ray Department, Luton & Dunstable Hospital NHS Trust, Lewsey Road, Luton, Beds LU4 0DZ, UK.

Leonie S. Paskin   Department of Radiology, Guy's Hospital, St Thomas Street, London SE1 9RT, UK.

Neil Prime   Department of Radiography, Canterbury Christ Church College, Canterbury, Kent CT1 1QU, UK.

Timothy Reynolds   Department of Radiographic Studies, North Staffordshire Hospital Centre, City General Hospital, Newcastle Road, Stoke-on-Trent ST4 6QG, UK.

Lynne Sterry   Division of Clinical Sciences, University of Hertfordshire, College Lane, Hatfield, Herts AL10 9AB, UK.

Josephine Swallow   Obstetrics and Gynaecology Ultrasound Department, Antenatal Clinic, University Hospital, Queens Medical Centre, Nottingham NG7 2UH, UK.

Andrew Todd-Pokropek   Medical Physics Department, University College London and Institute of Child Health, London WC1E 6AU, UK.

Elizabeth M. Warren   The MRI Centre, John Radcliffe Hospital, Headington, Oxford OX3 9DU, UK.

Cathy Williams   Centre for Cancer Treatment, Mount Vernon Hospital, Rickmansworth Road, Northwood, Middx HA6 2RN, UK.

Vivian Wood   Clinical Directorate of Neurology, The National Hospital for Neurology and Neurosurgery, Queen Square, London WC1N 3BG, UK.

Miles J. Woodford   X-ray Spinal Unit, Salisbury District General Hospital, Salisbury, Wilts SP2 8BJ, UK.

Judy Young   Lynda Jackson Macmillan Cancer Support and Information Centre, Mount Vernon Hospital, Rickmansworth Road, Northwood, Middx HA6 2RN, UK.

Preface

This first edition of *Current Topics in Radiography* arose from one of the many discussions that lamented the absence of a publication that focused specifically on developments occurring within radiography. A publication was needed which would provide a medium for practitioners to share experiences of the many changes taking place. In particular, we wanted to create an opportunity for new authors to come forward as well as inviting contributions from those with a wealth of experience in producing papers for professional and scientific publications. It was fortunate that W.B. Saunders Company were more than interested in the project and hence this first edition of *Current Topics*. Without the support of the publishers, the project would not have come to fruition and we are encouraged greatly that it is the intention to publish *Current Topics in Radiography* on an annual basis.

Our first task was to establish an editorial advisory panel to assist in identifying issues that would be topical and current at the time of publication. Potential authors were identified and approached. It was both gratifying and a relief to find that the great majority agreed, although some gentle encouragement had to be given in one or two cases! Authors were asked not to shy away from controversial matters and, when appropriate, to challenge traditional practices that have outlived their usefulness. After all, without controversy and challenge, which will sometimes be the cause of conflict, we cannot expect to move forwards. As well as controversies we wanted to include some leading-edge topics and cover the broad spectrum that makes up radiography. We are, therefore, especially grateful to the authors who contributed willingly to this first edition of *Current Topics*. We trust they will feel our editorial efforts have done justice to their contributions.

Publication coincides with the centenary celebrations of the discovery of X-rays. After one hundred years, radiography now encompasses the diagnostic and interventional modalities of x-ray imaging, ultrasound, radionuclide imaging and magnetic resonance imaging as well as radiotherapy and oncology. The centenary is celebrated at a time when radiography, both diagnostic and therapeutic, is undergoing profound change and the use of ionizing radiation for diagnosis and treatment is being questioned. It is appropriate, therefore, that we endeavour to record some of the current impacts on the profession in this new publication.

A final word to our readers: we hope that you will find that this book makes stimulating reading and that you will feel encouraged to contribute to future editions.

Audrey M. Paterson
Richard Price

1

Where Are We Now?

Olive M. Deaville

INTRODUCTION

Discussion of the professional status and role of radiographers produces varied views that reflect the major changes taking place within health care. Perceptions differ both within and outside radiography and are influenced by traditional attitudes and behaviour; however, there is acknowledgement that changes in roles and responsibilities are taking place (Department of Health, 1993). The most contentious issue relates to professional autonomy, which to date has been denied to radiographers within the clinical environment. Radiographers, their professional body, other professions, the Department of Health (DH) and the National Health Service Executive (NHSE) are the key players in this debate over the role of the radiographer and are driven by different motives in discussions about expanding these roles. The question 'Where are we now?' therefore produces some contradictory and conflicting views. These are presented here to stimulate further debate.

EDUCATION

Radiographers have gained academic qualifications and clinical competence by undergoing courses that have developed in breadth, depth and duration as the profession has responded to new technology and medical advances, for example, the diplomas in medical ultrasound and radionuclide imaging. Each change has been achieved because clinical radiographers have demonstrated their ability to learn new concepts and apply them in the practice of diagnosis and treatment. The achievement of degree status was earned by the recognition of this expertise, and with it came autonomy in education. The speed with which the basic qualification moved from diploma to degree was aided by government reforms (Department of Health, 1989), but can be credited to those within the profession who seized the opportunity (College of Radiographers, 1990a). This major educational change enabled radical revision of teaching and learning in both the academic and clinical arenas; the College of Radiographers (1990b) have published the criteria that would be applied in validating degree programmes.

The dilemma, for those responsible for education, is determining the role and responsibilities of the radiographers of tomorrow. First and second degrees that raise expectations of a greater role than is achievable may lead to frustration and a poorly motivated radiographer. Conversely, expanded knowledge and self-confidence may facilitate role development and enable the radiographer to practise as an autonomous professional.

The political climate continues to demand that the traditional pattern of health care provision is scrutinized and revised, and therefore the time is right for radiographers to be taking the lead in determining their future. Those involved in education need to join with clinical colleagues to ensure that this opportunity is not lost. Their combined vision of the future will inform members of the council of the professional body, the College of Radiographers, so enabling it to provide the leadership and support that the profession requires.

TECHNICAL AND SCIENTIFIC ABILITY

Advances in computerized imaging and radiotherapy equipment have been accompanied by a parallel expansion in the knowledge-base of radiographers. Their understanding of the scientific principles of new technologies has enabled them to play a leading role in image manipulation and treatment. The radiographer's role in the development of the practical application of new equipment is unique, and modifications and future developments are being made as a result of their informed dialogue with manufacturers. The next step will be for radiographers to become equal members of the research and development team.

There are several problems that need to be addressed before this involvement in research can take place. Radiographers need to show evidence that they have competence in research methods; this can be achieved through the study and research aspects of higher degrees. These courses of study are being undertaken by clinical radiographers, but support from their departments is given because there is an expectation that the outcome will be of direct benefit to that service. A radiographer who gains these qualifications may meet with obstacles if they then wish to undertake full-time research. A secondment to a university or manufacturer, for a stated period of time, would ensure that the individual could return to the clinical department without a break in service. This may not gain support, and therefore resignation and re-employment may be the only option. This may be detrimental financially as research posts can be less favourably rewarded than a National Health Service (NHS) post. Research posts often offer only short-term contracts and will result in a break in service and a gap in clinical experience, which may mean that return to an NHS post may be difficult. Full-time research may only be possible for those employed in the education sector unless individual terms and conditions can be negotiated with the trust hospital.

For those radiographers who leave the NHS there is an additional problem that relates to their professional status. It is probable that in their research role they are not designated as radiographers and therefore begin to question the benefits of retaining membership of the Society and College of Radiographers. The trade union may no longer be able to represent them in the workplace and the professional support they require can be obtained elsewhere. They cease membership and, as a consequence, these radiographers are lost to the profession and the outcome of their research is published and credited elsewhere.

INTERPERSONAL, COMMUNICATION AND MANAGEMENT SKILLS

The environment in which radiographers work is composed of many different staff groups with various skills and qualifications. In order for the service to function efficiently, good interpersonal skills are required. Radiographers have taken the lead in recognizing this and gain valuable experience in general management whilst practising in the clinical department. When these interpersonal and communication skills are given the opportunity to develop, radiographers have shown their ability to manage staff and significant financial budgets. In the values, beliefs and skills if the concept of the multidisciplinary team is to triumph for the common good of patients. The days of one profession dominating another have no place at the end of the twentieth century. The stakeholders in radiography are radiographers and it is a responsibility incumbent upon radiographers to develop new skills relevant to practice in a multidisciplinary workplace. The extended role is promoted by the College of Radiographers (1994) and is achievable within the Statement of Conduct issued by the Radiographers Board (1993). But let there be no doubt that autonomy demands total responsibility for their actions from those who seek it.

References

College of Radiographers (1990a) *Radiography Education and Training for the Future: A New Policy*. London: College of Radiographers.

College of Radiographers (1990b) *The Development of Degree Courses: A Handbook*. London: College of Radiographers.

College of Radiographers (1994) *Code of Professional Conduct*. London: College of Radiographers.

Department of Health/College of Radiographers (1993) *Imaging Department Skill Mix Study*. London: Her Majesty's Stationery Office.

Department of Health (1989) *Working for Patients: Education and Training (Working Paper 10)*. London: Her Majesty's Stationery Office.

Radiographers' Board of the Council for the Professions Supplementary to Medicine (1993) *Statement of Conduct*. London: Council for the Professions Supplementary to Medicine.

2

The Future of Ionizing Radiation Medicine in Diagnosis and Therapy

Elizabeth J. McLean

INTRODUCTION

The use of ionizing radiation for medical purposes is quoted as the largest man-made contribution to the UK population dose (Hughes et al., 1989). In an up-date on the frequency of x-ray examinations in Great Britain (Wall et al., 1986), the annual total of examinations was estimated to be 35 million, representing an average increase of 2% per annum since the first estimates made. Hicks (1993) demonstrated that public perception of radiation risk underestimates the actual risk incurred. Articles in recent journals indicate the need for increased control of the use of ionizing radiation and promote the use of protocols and systems of good practice in order to reduce both the unnecessary use of radiation and the waste of costly resources.

The three main areas of focus within this chapter are radiology, nuclear medicine and radiotherapy over the next 20 years. The effects of changes in ultrasound practice and magnetic resonance imaging will be referred to where they impinge on the changes within the other disciplines. In all areas the future will evolve around changes in technology, techniques, the operating environment and case mix.

OPERATING ENVIRONMENT

A recent National Association of Health Authorities and Trusts (NAHAT) report looking beyond the next decade suggested there would be fewer than 30 acute hospitals and an emphasis on health promotion and care in the community. The emphasis on value for money in a cash-limited industry will clearly continue to impact on decision-making processes. Responsibility for the purchase of health-care, technology and skills will be devolved fully to general practitioner (GP) purchasers, either directly or indirectly. The return of community-style hospitals in the guise of polyclinics, or facilities with primary-care beds managed by GPs, is envisaged by some. Paterson (1994b) cites that many diagnostic imaging examinations will be carried out in community- or primary-care settings. This would allow patients to attend the relevant secondary/tertiary centre with a definitive diagnosis or when a complex diagnosis or treatment schedule is required, as proposed for example in *A Policy Framework for Commissioning Cancer Services* (Consultative Document, 1994).

Care in the Community

It is envisaged that physicians could examine their patients and, when necessary, carry out their own imaging immediately. Hussain (1994) demonstrates that some training in ultrasound is already beginning for this purpose. Alternatively, community-based premises could have a multi-skilled 'technician' available to carry out a variety of tasks. These could include imaging, taking blood and preparing slides, counselling, advising on treatment options, and liaising with colleagues in the secondary centres. Some GPs have installed x-ray equipment in their practices in the UK, although Evans (1993) notes that in-house facilities are uncommon in the USA, as indeed they are in Europe. A number of facilities are already available on a sessional basis through mobile services, with or without professional back-up, and this looks set to expand.

Many radiologists find these ideas untenable and do not consider peripatetic or community-based radiographers, physicians or surgeons performing radiological functions acceptable from the perspectives of cost, quality and professional protection. Hopper et al. (1991) indicate the problems, and potentially serious consequences, of inadequate marking and reporting of chest radiographs by non-radiologists with little experience and where throughput is very low.

Role Changes for All Professionals

The implementation of the Calman Report (Calman, 1993) will have a major impact on the organization of services and the roles and responsibilities of doctors. The impact of fewer trainees receiving shorter, more intensive training which is knowledge rather than experience based (as is currently the case) will lead to fewer, less experienced physicians in senior positions. It will increase the pressure on medical staff who will be required both to train such juniors and themselves provide the clinical service rather than lead it. In addition, the absence of an increased budget to employ additional consultants to spread the load and the inability to recruit easily given fewer potential applicants will combine to create an intolerable situation. This must lead to changes in perception about who is the most appropriate person to take on specific roles and tasks (Smy, 1994).

Re-engineering of systems and procedures is already taking place along with analysis of roles and responsibilities in preparation for local pay bargaining. Audits of radiographer-based ultrasound services, performance of barium enemas, injections of contrast agents, and reporting of radiographs broach the subject of boundary shifts between professionals and demonstrate acceptability, accuracy and perceived benefits (Saxton, 1992; Weston et al., 1994; Staab and Stewart, 1994; British Institute of Radiology, 1994). It is perceived that there is a role for radiotherapy radiographers to plan, monitor, adjust fields as necessary and hold treatment-review clinics. Medical time will be more devoted to interventional procedures than diagnostic processes, and it is thought possible that radiologists and nuclear medicine technologists will hold diagnostic clinics, have their own bed allocations and receive tertiary referrals (Kimber, 1994).

Service Changes

In secondary centres in particular, customer demand for far more accessibility, the need for effective, efficient and intensive use of high-cost plant, and alterations to treatment patterns will require the extension of the working day and implementation of a standard 7-day week (Hately, 1993). This would be facilitated by the envisaged changes in roles and responsibilities. In the meantime, it is resisted strongly by some in all disciplines.

At the local- or community-hospital level, 'basic' imaging, data transfer and some treatments will be undertaken, thereby removing this

3

Are Radiologists Really Necessary?

Anthony R. Divers

INTRODUCTION

The first century since the discovery of X-rays has seen exciting developments in medical imaging, the formation of the centralized radiology department and the increasing monopoly of medical radiology by radiologists. The impact on and the benefit to patient care from medical imaging is incalculable. This is not a static position and new developments and technology will continue, probably at a greater pace than previously. But what of the radiologist? Several factors (Table 3.1) have influenced, and will continue to influence the role of the radiologist and the radiographer. This chapter will explore these factors.

The pessimistic scenario for radiologists is that, although new techniques and technologies will keep medical imaging in a pivotal position of patient care, the role of the radiologist will become superfluous. Surgeons and physicians, aided by new computer systems that enable the display and storage of images which they can interpret themselves,

Table 3.1 Factors influencing the role of the radiologist

Historic development of medical imaging
NHS management reforms
Radiological workload
New technology and techniques
The expanding role of other imaging professionals

together with new technology and techniques and the pressure from National Health Service (NHS) managers, will no longer refer patients to the clinical radiologist.

HISTORY OF THE DEVELOPMENT OF MEDICAL IMAGING

The medical value of X-rays was realized rapidly by the scientific community following the announcement of their discovery by Professor Wilhelm Conrad Röntgen in the *Annals of the Medical Society of Wursburg* in 1895 (Röntgen, 1895). In the UK the first published photograph of a medical X-ray was in 1896 in the *British Medical Journal* by A. Campbell Swinton (Campbell Swinton, 1896), an electrical engineer. The history of who should control the X-ray tube, its directions and the interpretation of the resultant image is fascinating, and key dates and events are shown in Table 3.2.

Table 3.2   The history of the medical monopoly of the X-ray tube

1895	Discovery of X-rays by Röntgen at the University of Wursburg
1896	First printed photograph of an X-ray in UK (Campbell Swinton, *British Medical Journal*)
	Medical imaging in the UK is born
	Only plain-film radiographs
1896	First radiological journal published in the UK
1897	Röntgen Society formed
1904	Rieder–Bismuth contrast media for gastrointestinal-tract imaging
1917	British Association for the Advancement of Radiology and Physiotherapy formed
1920	First Diploma in Radiology (BAARP)
	Society of Radiographers formed
1924	British Institute of Radiology formed
1930	Thorotrast Vascular Radiology introduced
1936	Society of Radiographers becomes a founder member of the Board of Regulation of Medical Auxiliaries
1939	Faculty of Radiology formed
1940s	Water-soluble contrast media become available
1951	Cope Committee recommendations on qualifications for NHS radiographers
1970s	Computed tomography introduced
1985	The Ionizing Radiation Regulations introduced
1988	Protection of Persons undergoing Medical Examinations and Treatment Regulations introduced
1990s	Rapid growth of magnetic resonance imaging

The development of the monopoly of medical imaging by radiologists parallels the advancement in radiological technology and the realization of the dangers of radiation exposure (Larkin, 1983). The first days of medical imaging involved plain-film examination of bones, joints and the chest, and the localization of foreign bodies. Hospitals often employed engineers or lay radiographers (unqualified radiographers) to provide X-ray imaging services, since they invariably owned the machines and the physicians and surgeons of the day had no wish for competition from clinical radiologists. Societies for doctors, lay radiographers and engineers formed and produced their own journals and, as the complexity and clinical usefulness of medical imaging grew and the risks of radiation were learned, the processes of regulation, training and qualification commenced. By 1924, rulings from the Board of Trade and the General Medical Council prohibited the lay radiographer and engineer from directing the radiographic exposure. In 1936, the Board of Regulation of Medical Auxiliaries, later to become the Council for Professions Supplementary to Medicine, was formed with the Society of Radiographers as a founder member, and the medical monopoly was complete. In 1951 the Cope Committee recommended that the Diploma of Radiography be a pre-condition of employment for radiographers in NHS hospitals.

The Ionizing Radiation Regulations and associated guidelines of the 1980s (National Radiological Protection Board, 1988) correctly identified and enshrined the need for those personnel who direct and control ionizing radiation examinations or treatments to be trained and qualified persons. No specific role is enshrined for the radiologist, and the ultimate responsibility for providing protective measures lies with the employer who may be a company, an NHS Health Authority or Board, an NHS Trust, or a self-employed person such as a general practitioner (GP) in a group practice.

NHS MANAGEMENT CHANGES

The NHS management reforms have brought, and continue to bring, great change to the provision of health care in the UK. The term 'reform' is inappropriate, as it implies that something was irrefutably wrong with the service and that the reforms have 'improved' the situation. The purchaser–provider split, the formation of NHS Trusts and the increasing purchasing power of fundholder GPs have resulted in review and scrutiny of medical practice, including medical imaging, with the prominence of 'cost' issues. Radiologists are well trained but expensive. Is it good value for money for radiologists to report every plain film (Emrys-Roberts, 1975), or to undertake routine ultrasound examinations? What about the bulk of routine screening examinations and intravenous urograms? Dermatologists do not see every patient in their district with a rash. Only when primary care runs into problems is specialist advice sought. The routine obstetric ultrasound service is predominantly served by ultrasonographers, and as the general ultrasound workload increases, so will the pressure to allow this area to be passed over to an increasingly ultrasonographer-led service. Name a hospital able to provide an open access, radiologist-run ultrasound service!

The pressures on the medical imaging service are immense, and if radiologists are to survive, and not to be cut back like dead wood, then they must mark out their role as the 'conductor of the orchestra' (Carty, 1994), directing imaging and investigations in the most appropriate way, and supervising the increasing areas of medical imaging performed by radiographers. Are radiologists to become extinct as dinosaurs, or to survive as mammals?

RADIOLOGICAL WORKLOAD

The Royal College of Radiologists has drawn attention to the increase in workload in clinical radiology (Royal College of Radiologists, 1993). Between 1968 and 1991 the total workload trebled, but during the same period of time the number of radiologists in NHS posts in England and Wales only doubled. A comparison with other Western countries shows the relatively low number of radiologists in the UK, but a fairly average rate of use of radiology. This disparity between workload and the number of radiologists will continue to increase, probably at a greater rate. Pressures of the competitive market may lead to a view of efficiency as more work for less money, with shorter waiting times as the quality issue.

There is no sign of additional funding to close the gap between workload and the number of radiologists, and stark choices face current working practices and standards in medical imaging. But who will set the standards? Radiologists must be prepared to face these challenges and must initiate new working practices involving radiographers. They must set new standards and provide real value for money. Clinical audit will be the vehicle used to evaluate these new standards.

3. Radiology nursing staff were often called to deal with these minor reactions.

Since the radiographers have taken on this role, audit has revealed a number of advantages:

1. Reduced waiting time for the patient.
2. Reduced levels of stress for the patient.
3. Improved continuity of care.
4. Reduction in adverse reactions experienced by the patient.
5. Radiology nursing staff rarely called to assist.

It may be concluded that the introduction of radiographers to the administration of intravenous injections has presented no problems and has in fact benefited both the patient and the department. A radiologist supervises each intravenous urogram session and is available for support and advice if this is required. Support is sometimes required regarding the film sequence relevant to the patient's clinical history, but rarely regarding the intravenous injection.

IDENTIFICATION OF ABNORMALITIES BY RADIOGRAPHERS

In 1988, the superintendent radiographer in charge of the accident service X-ray department, supported by the consultant radiologists and the consultant in charge of the accident service department, started to assess the feasibility of radiographers identifying abnormalities demonstrated on the films undertaken in accident service X-ray. Any suspected abnormality was to be indicated by placing a red spot on the film.

When first discussed with the radiographic staff, some hesitancy was expressed about the scheme. However, the superintendent radiographer in charge of accident service X-ray had decided to undertake her HDCR Module F project on this topic, and hence the radiographic staff willingly agreed to participate, to enable this project to be completed. Once underway, radiographers began to take much more interest in the anatomical and pathological details on the films, which stimulated much discussion about suspected abnormalities and the need for additional projections to demonstrate these fully.

Junior medical staff were encouraged to discuss films with the radiographers concerned, particularly if the reason for placing a red spot on the film was not obvious. This resulted in improved communications between the radiographers and junior medical staff.

Medico-legal aspects needed to be considered. Radiographers are covered by the College of Radiographers Code of Professional Conduct and the Radiographers Board statement on this aspect of the extended role. There was also an agreement locally to support these working practices and the director of radiology formally communicated these to the chief executive and the consultant in charge of accident service.

It was necessary to highlight the following points to the junior medical staff:

1. The red spot is an informal signal from the radiographer to the casualty officer, based on the radiographic and practical experience of the radiographer concerned. It is not a definitive diagnosis and should not be treated as such. The legal and professional responsibility for the initial assessment of the radiograph lies with the casualty officer.
2. The absence of a red dot does not imply that the X-ray is normal, but simply that the radiographer has not identified any abnormality on it.

It was recognized that training and audit were the key to the success of this project, and therefore these were monitored from the beginning.

Tutorials, where trauma films were discussed, were held for the radiographers by a consultant radiologist and the consultant in charge of accident service. Radiographers now participate in the orthopaedic meetings which are held regularly and where interesting cases are discussed and interchange of ideas takes place.

Three audit surveys were undertaken which involved monitoring the x-ray films of 500 patients whose examinations were considered normal by the senior house officers in the accident service department.

In the first survey, 500 sets of radiographs considered normal by the senior house officers in the accident service were reported by radiologists who discovered 33 abnormalities. This represented a 6.6% diagnostic failure rate.

In the second survey, radiographers indicated (by means of a code on the request form) those radiographs which they considered showed an abnormality. Medical staff in the accident service were not made aware of this. Five hundred sets of radiographs considered normal by the junior medical staff were reported by the radiologists who discovered

26 abnormalities (5.2%). Fourteen of these had been identified as abnormal by the radiographers.

In the third survey, the radiographers were asked to put a red spot on the films that they considered to be abnormal, prior to the films being seen by the junior medical staff. After the 'red spotting' system commenced, 500 normal sets of radiographs were reported by the radiologist. Twelve abnormalities were discovered (2.4%).

The audit therefore demonstrated that the red spot system reduced the number of abnormalities missed by the junior medical staff. The red spot system works well and is now part of departmental life. Since the introduction of this system a greater number of abnormalities have been detected at the first assessment than were previously.

The main problem from the radiographic viewpoint is that radiographers tend to 'over spot', thereby producing false positives. This is probably due to the large number of radiographers, of varying levels of experience, who are rostered through accident service, thus causing a variation in the standard of assessment.

This system could well be extended further to progress the role of the radiographer. Experienced radiographers could undertake a 'first read' of accident films, separating those films that require a radiological opinion from those that do not. A trial of radiographers undertaking a 'first read' of accident films commenced in March 1995. Formal training of radiographic staff and some increase in resources will be required to implement such a system on a long term basis.

BARIUM ENEMAS

In 1993, a decision was taken to extend the role of the radiographer by allowing radiographers to conduct barium enema examinations. Two senior II radiographers were selected to undertake this training.

Formal authorization was obtained in writing from the clinical director of radiology. The chief executive was also informed, in writing, that radiographers were to undertake barium enema examinations. The trained radiographers have been issued with, and work to, a protocol which is based on the one developed by St James' University Hospital, Leeds.

The two selected radiographers attended the training course organized by St James' University Hospital, Leeds. On the recommendation of the course organizers the supervising consultant radiologist also attended the first part of the course. This was invaluable as he was made aware of the aims and objectives of the course and the training provided. The consultant was very supportive in establishing this procedure at departmental level, in assisting with protocols, and in acting as an advocate for the trained radiographers.

The course at St James consisted of:

1. 1.5 days of theory – topics covered included film sequence, contraindications, complications, pathology, bowel preparation, pharmacology of antispasmodics.
2. One-day refresher course.

The course proved excellent, providing a firm theoretical basis. The radiographers returned after the introductory part of the course fired with enthusiasm and eager to start.

Initially the two trained radiographers worked together when undertaking barium enemas, benefiting from the mutual encouragement and support. They now work with other radiographers, forming part of an in-house training programme.

The procedure for a radiographer-conducted barium enema examination is as follows:

1. Request forms are vetted by the supervising radiologist. The prescribed dose of antispasmodic is written on the request form.
2. The patient's medical history is checked for any contraindications to the prescribed antispasmodic.
3. Patient preparation procedures are checked.
4. Intravenous injection of the antispasmodic is given by the radiographer.
5. Barium is run into the large bowel under screening control. The patient is turned and gas insufflated to produce double-contrast images.
6. The films are shown to the supervising radiologist once the standard sequence has been obtained. Additional projections are taken by the radiographer or radiologist, as appropriate. The supervising radiologist can be called during the procedure if required.

Audit of the procedure has been undertaken and has revealed the following:

1. There has been a reduction in the length of the barium enema waiting list. Radiographers undertook 350 barium enema examinations between April 1993 and July 1994.
2. No delay is experienced by the patient at the commencement of the

examination, as the radiographer is on hand. Radiologists are often covering more than one area of the department and are therefore not always immediately available.

3. Continuity of care is improved as the person undertaking the examination is present throughout the procedure.
4. Screening times were initially longer, but are now comparable with those of the radiologists.
5. Radiographers work to an agreed protocol when taking the films. On average, radiographers take three more films per patient than do the radiologists.
6. Films taken are of a higher technical quality.
7. Radiological time is reduced and, therefore, other work can be performed by the radiologist while the barium enema lists are progressing.
8. Immediate feedback on the outcome of the examination cannot be given to the patient. Feedback is often expected and desirable for the patient's peace of mind and would seem to be the main disadvantage of radiographers undertaking barium enema examinations.

The radiographic staff involved in undertaking barium enema examinations enjoy this aspect of their role extension. Since the scheme has been introduced it has ensured more effective use of limited radiological resources.

ULTRASOUND

Ultrasound was one of the first areas where role extension took place. It is now commonplace and the norm in most departments for radiographers to scan patients and issue their own reports. Therefore, in this chapter only a brief outline is given of this role.

Formal approval is given in writing by the chief executive for sonographers to scan and issue reports on obstetric, gynaecological and general cases. Individual authorization is given to each sonographer, in writing, by the consultant obstetrician and radiologist responsible for ultrasound scanning.

Good diploma and, more recently, MSc courses exist for training radiographers in ultrasound and, over the years, we have used these courses to train sonographers. Liaison takes place between the clinical establishments and training organizations to ensure that theoretical knowledge is supported by clinical aptitude and expertise. Encouragingly, some training establishments are now including clinical assessment at departmental level as part of the final qualification process. Therefore, if a sonographer is not competent clinically they will fail the final examination.

In obstetric and gynaecological ultrasound, sonographers undertake and issue a report on all scans, using the vaginal approach where appropriate. On completion of the scan the sonographer discusses outcomes with the patient, with support from the appropriate medical team and nurse counsellor when required. Tertiary referrals are made by the sonographers to other centres if complex fetal abnormalities are diagnosed. These referrals are made for assessment of prognosis, implications of certain diagnosed conditions and also for genetic studies. Recent referrals have included:

1. Fetal anomaly of the bowel (Hirschsprung's disease).
2. Complex chromosome abnormality.

Close liaison, and mutual respect, exists between the sonographers and the obstetric and gynaecological medical teams. There is ongoing participation of the sonographers in the regular clinical meetings, with the sonographers presenting case studies regularly.

Audit forms part of the daily routine, with interesting cases logged and followed up for outcome. This leads to a more formal audit being undertaken to show the effectiveness of routine ultrasonography in detecting fetal structural abnormalities in a district general hospital. We have shown that routine ultrasonography by sonographers in a low-risk population is effective in detecting many structural malformations (Chitty et al., 1991).

Direct comparison with other studies is difficult because they do not include details of the less severe abnormalities. However, our results, detecting 74.4% of all abnormalities in the screened population and 71.5% in the total population, compare favourably with other reports (detection of major anomalies 39.4–83%) (Saari-Kemppainen et al., 1990).

THE FUTURE

With the introduction of graduate staff and the research base that is being established in the profession, the climate is right to extend the role of the radiographer further. Degree courses are providing students with the strong theoretical base that will be required to facilitate this.

However, at post-diploma/graduate level there is still a lack of appropriate training courses for aspects of the extended role. Teaching and clinical staff must continue to work together to ensure that correct training is provided. This must include regular update and refresher courses for aspects of the extended role, with consideration given to some of these becoming mandatory, for example, on a 5-yearly basis.

At departmental level, training, money and appropriate resources are crucial for progression of the extended role. This must be accompanied by appropriate remuneration of staff which is consistent with the additional responsibility.

In-house training, film viewing, and meetings between relevant disciplines should become a normal part of departmental life, thereby ensuring regular exchange of ideas and ongoing training.

CONCLUSION

The extended role of the radiographer at Luton & Dunstable Hospital NHS Trust is firmly established and an everyday part of departmental life. Radiographers have proven that they are eager and able to extend their role. When given the authority and opportunity to do so, they undertake this to a high standard with greater attention to detail. Job satisfaction, motivation and professional confidence have increased. The success of these changes has been dependent upon correct selection and training of staff and the continued support of the consultant radiological staff.

COMMENT Audrey M. Paterson, *Canterbury*

The Luton & Dunstable NHS Trust is to be congratulated in the progress it has made in developing the roles of its radiographers. Clearly, the trust began this work some considerable time ago and is likely to be in the forefront of radiographic practice. However, it could be argued that the approach has been task oriented and somewhat piecemeal, based largely on the drives of reducing resources and increasing demands. What appears to be lacking is a fundamental review of the potential roles and functions of all staff groups within the radiology department relative to the changing priorities and demands being made on the department. Luton & Dunstable NHS Trust is not alone in this. Most other trusts engaging in radiographic role-development activities are taking the task-centred approach.

In considering the role developments that have taken place at Luton & Dunstable, it becomes apparent that radiographers have adopted new, and extended, practices well. But these do not appear to be moving on. For example, radiographers now give intravenous injections of contrast media – yet they still require the supervision and support of a radiologist, particularly in relation to the film sequences needed in relation to patients' clinical histories. It is somewhat of a paradox that radiographers, whose prime function has always been the radiographic examination, should require such support but need it only 'rarely' in relation to the intravenous injection of contrast media – a relatively new and so-called 'extended' function of radiographers.

There are other examples where role extension has not yet led to role development. The red spot system has been in operation since 1988. It has been audited and has been found to be helpful. It has also been suggested that the scheme could be extended further so that experienced radiographers undertake a first-read, or screen, of films to identify those that require a radiological opinion. This would, indeed, be further development of the red spot system in operation, but is it enough? Could not a case be made for radiographers to be developed so that they make written reports on all examinations they carry out? This would provide what are often junior medical staff with clear, unambiguous information and a radiograph – no longer would they have to wonder why a red spot had been attached to a film or worry when there was no red spot on a radiograph which they felt was abnormal. Yes, the red spot system is a highly commendable example of role development in radiography, but it could be so much more.

Similarly, role extension into barium enema examinations and into ultrasound imaging needs to become real development and some of the current constraints need to be questioned. Why does a radiographer need to take more films during a barium enema than does a radiologist? Why can immediate feedback about a radiographer-conducted barium enema not be given to the patient? Why is there a distinction in the nature of radiographers' practice between obstetric and gynaecological ultrasound imaging and general abdominal scanning?

There are no simple, or single, answers to these questions. However, if role extension – the task-oriented approach to changing practice – is to become both a quantitative and a qualitative leap in radiographic practice and, hence, true development, then these questions must be addressed. Luton & Dunstable NHS Trust have a excellent basis from which to begin tackling them.

Acknowledgements

To all the staff in the Imaging Directorate at Luton & Dunstable Hospital NHS Trust, whose work is detailed in this article.

References

Chitty, L., Hunt, G., Moore, J. et al. (1991) Effectiveness of routine ultra-sonography in detecting fetal structural abnormalities in a low risk population. *British Medical Journal* **303:** 1165–1169.

Saari-Kemppainen, A., Karjalainen, O., Ylostalo, P. et al. (1990) Ultrasound screening and perinatal mortality: controlled trial of systematic one-stage screening in pregnancy. *Lancet* **336:** 387–391.

5

Patient Focus in Radiography – the Challenges

Diane Carney

INTRODUCTION

The competitive environment of the health-care market has encouraged many National Health Service (NHS) Trust hospitals to review and develop services which meet the demands of their customers – primarily the patient, the general practitioner (GP) and the health authority. It is essential that trust hospitals retain and gain purchaser contracts in order to survive as a viable health-care unit. To gain and maintain the competitive edge they must maximize all resources and ensure that the services they provide are of a higher quality than previously, with little or no extra cost to the purchaser. Hence, provider units must seek improvements to existing services and must introduce new policies and procedures to increase efficiency and the standard of care.

In 1991, the National Health Service Management Executive (NHSME) offered sponsorship and support to seven trust pilot sites in the UK for the development and research of a new care concept which would increase efficiency and improve the quality of care. The care concept was identified as the 'patient-focused' or 'patient-centred' approach.

The patient-focused approach was originally developed in the USA to address issues relating to patient care by assuring that care is centred or focused around the needs of the patient. Implementation of the patient-focused approach presents many challenges to health-care professionals as it involves changing the highly hierarchical and bureaucratic organizational culture of NHS hospitals. The patient-focus approach thus identified several restructuring principles which, when invoked, focus care around patients' needs.

One restructuring principle suggests moving services closer to the patient's bedside. The decentralization of diagnostic services such as radiology to autonomous patient-focus units has raised many professional issues and created endless debate as to the benefits and challenges of introducing the patient-focus concept.

THE PATIENT-FOCUSED CARE CONCEPT

Management consultants examining trust hospital pilot sites discovered similar patterns in patient care by examining the service as through the eyes of a patient. Booz-Allen and Hamilton, management consultants (1991), found inpatient care at one of the pilot sites to be:

1. Marked by delays (to get in, while in, and to get out).
2. Fragmented, discontinuous and depersonalized ('a procession of faces').
3. Lacking a single point of accountability and information.
4. An unplanned adventure for patients and staff.
5. Provided by the least trained staff and staff in training.
6. Remote from senior management.

The patient-focus approach is designed to address these very issues by radically changing the organizational culture. Attitudes, procedures and systems of work must be changed to focus on patient needs and the improvement of care.

Most NHS hospitals are highly compartmentalized and functionally oriented. The majority of staff groups are health-care professionals who frequently demonstrate job overspecification. There is a high degree of task demarcation and low accountability and, as a result, fragmentation of patient care within hospital units.

The patient-focus concept identifies a number of restructuring principles which should be implemented to address patient-care issues. These principles have, and will, create a number of challenges to all health-care professionals involved in developing the concept. The patient-focus restructuring principles, as identified by Booz-Allen and Hamilton in 1991, were:

1. *Place patient services closer to the bedside.* This includes diagnostic and therapeutic, as well as management, clerical and support services.
2. *Multiskill staff to broaden capabilities.* Development of a wide range of care skills shared by all team members. All team members to be trained in core duties, for example, issuing bedpans, lifting and handling, administration of food and drink.
3. *Develop self-sufficient patient-care teams.* These will care for small groups of patients, providing continuity of care so that 90% of patient-care delivery is from within a patient-care team. This involvement of all staff in patient care will increase the time spent on direct care giving.
4. *Integrate demand management and scheduling.* This could be achieved by: simplifying processes; by reducing the number of work-steps and number of staff involved in each of the processes; and by improving scheduling, particularly lengths of stays, admissions and discharges.
5. *Use patient protocols and critical paths to manage care.* Develop standard integrated plans for entire stays, for example, a myocardial infarct (MI) patient protocol. Reduce documentation by using computerized case notes and protocol software, and charting by exception. Set quality standards for care, and underpin with clinical audit.

For the purpose of this chapter, the first and second principles have been examined to determine the challenges they create for the central radiology and medical-imaging departments within those hospitals whose management choose the patient-focus care route.

Restructuring Principle 1: To Move Services Closer to the Patient's Bedside

Placement of services nearer to the patient's bedside involves the decentralization of core diagnostic services such as those of radiology and pathology. It is evident that centralized radiology departments and pathology units have remained and have continued to grow over the past two decades. There are two main reasons for this. Firstly, the proliferation and continued development of imaging techniques and technologies. Secondly, the commonly held understanding that high-capital-cost equipment should be fully utilized to justify expenditure of public health funds.

The cost of developing and running a satellite radiographic unit would involve initial purchase costs of a general-purpose radiographic unit, processing equipment, accessories and building enabling work. Running costs would include staffing, equipment-service contracts, overheads, training, equipment depreciation costs and capital charges. Capital charges are the notional rate of return that hospitals are required to deliver on the equipment and land they use.

Advocates of the patient-focus approach argue that centralization to achieve economies of scale within the NHS has resulted in a situation where an increased number of operational steps have been introduced into the care process. As a consequence, funds are not being entirely spent on the medical, technical and clinical aspects of patient care, but rather on arranging it, documenting it, and on waiting for it to happen. The introduction of the patient-focus approach through development of a satellite radiography unit would reduce process time and re-emphasize direct patient care. It may also identify variable cost savings on staff time which would counter capital charges and depreciation costs.

It must be recognized at this point that the amount of diagnostic X-ray procedures carried out within a patient-focus satellite radiographic unit will vary greatly, depending on the local geography, the hospital's systems of work, the types of patient utilizing the unit, for example, orthopaedic patients, medical or geriatric patients and, most significantly, the existing organizational culture.

Restructuring Principle 2: Multiskill Staff to Broaden Capabilities

The patient-focus approach encourages staff involvement and ownership through the removal of compartmentalization of attitudes, and certain professional boundaries. The team approach has many potential benefits. However, the issue of multiskilling can be a contentious one. It is therefore crucial that cross-boundary professional training is sensitive to the needs of individual professions and must maintain the necessary professional standards and regulations to provide a safe, high standard of service. The patient-focus approach does not remove the need for professional, expert knowledge. The contention is whether these professional skills can be deployed safely in a different environment and as part of a team approach to patient care.

Patient-focus hospital units encouraging health-care workers other than state-registered radiographers to carry out diagnostic X-ray examinations may contravene NHS regulations implicated by the Professions Supplementary to Medicine Act, 1960, and the Ionizing

Radiations Regulations (1985, 1988). Staff employed in the NHS from the professions supplementary to medicine (chiropodists, dieticians, medical laboratory scientific officers, occupational therapists, orthoptists, physiotherapists and radiographers) are required to be state registered by an approved statutory body – in the case of radiographers, the Radiographers Board of the Council for Professions Supplementary to Medicine (CPSM).

To utilize state-registered staff time more effectively and increase the staff time spent on the medical, technical and clinical aspects of patient care, it is necessary to multiskill individual professionals in other less complicated skills such as phlebotomy, electrocardiography (ECG) and basic nursing skills such as bed-making, lifting and feeding of patients. It is essential that the training and supervision of these areas is comprehensive, on-going and to an agreed, assessed, professional level of competence. It can be argued that involvement in numerous non-radiographic tasks may counter any time savings due to the non-availability of the patient-focus radiographer when undertaking these other cross-trained duties. Low volumes of inpatient radiographic duties may also result in the dilution of the patient-focus radiographer's more expert radiographic skills.

THE BENEFITS OF DEVELOPING AN INPATIENT PATIENT-FOCUS RADIOLOGY UNIT

The patient-focus team approach to care claims many benefits for the patient, the central radiology department and to the patient-focus unit staff.

Benefits to the Inpatient

1. *Personalized service*: the patient is able to build a relationship with the unit radiographer which increases the patient's trust and confidence in the service.
2. *Increased privacy and dignity*: the patient will not suffer the indignity of a, possibly, long journey to the central department in their night attire. They will no longer endure a long wait in an often exposed, cold waiting area.
3. *Reduced x-ray appointment times*: the unit radiographer will be more accessible to vet and discuss requests for X-ray examinations. These requests will no longer have to wait to be sent to the central

department at the convenience of ward clerks or junior medical officers. This will reduce the process time and patients will be examined sooner. The overall reduction in appointment times could be instrumental in the reduction of the patient's length of stay within the patient-focus unit. X-ray appointments will be co-ordinated by the unit radiographer more effectively and arranged at times more convenient to other patient-focus team staff. Hence patients would not forego any other treatment to attend an x-ray appointment, for example, physiotherapy treatment or dietary advice.

4. *Continuous care*: a multiskilled radiographer will be able to carry out an increased number of diagnostic tests at any one appointment time, for example, an ECG, a chest x-ray or phlebotomy. If the tests are carried out by a single radiographer and subsequently recorded, confidence that the tests had been carried out would be increased and hence lessen the chance of their unnecessary duplication.

5. *Patient knowledge*: a patient-focus unit radiographer would develop a closer working relationship with patients as part of the patient-focus care team. The unit radiographer would spend a greater amount of time directly explaining and informing the patients about medical-imaging procedures, and also in allaying any patient concerns and fears.

6. *Correct patient preparation*: development of effective communication will ensure that there is less risk of patients receiving incorrect or inadequate preparation prior to specialized radiology procedures, for example, eating prior to a barium meal investigation. Accurate patient preparation will result in a reduction of abandoned examinations, re-testing and subsequent delays in patient disease diagnosis.

Benefits to the Central Radiology Department

1. *Effective communication*: the patient-focus unit radiographer will provide an essential communication link with the central radiology department. The patient-focus unit radiographer will become the central point of contact. The radiographer could readily exchange information between the unit and the central department. This would reduce the time wasted by radiology department staff contacting a range and number of ward staff by telephone, and minimize staff time spent issuing patient-preparation instructions.

2. *Reduced cancelled/abandoned special examinations*: involvement of the radiographer in the patient-focus unit team would ensure that fewer X-ray examinations are abandoned or unnecessarily

extended through the incorrect preparation of patients and malassessment of patients' conditions, for example, physical disabilities, asthma and diabetes.

3. *Effective use of radiology personnel*: radiology department staff would spend less time arranging transport, acquiring previous x-ray films and answering patient-focus unit queries. Less time would be spent waiting for the often delayed arrival of patient-focus unit patients for general radiographic procedures.

4. *Efficient radiology workload management*: there would be a reduced number of inpatients examined within the central department. Inpatients generally require a greater length of examination time due to their degree of illness. Hence, the central department will be able to maximize the resultant spare operational capacity, either by introducing new services for GPs, for example, walk-in services, or by enabling a greater degree of flexibility in existing services to ensure that GP Patient Charter standards are achieved.

Benefits to Patient-focus Unit Staff

1. *Job enrichment*: staff who become multiskilled in a variety of clinical areas may enrich their present roles. Job enrichment will reduce the monotony and boredom of routine, often mundane, tasks. As a result, job motivation may also be increased when staff are recognized for more tasks and when they understand the significance of their actions in relation to the success of the overall patient care.

2. *Job satisfaction*: spending more time with patients by carrying out a variety of tests will enable the patient-focus unit radiographer to chart the progress of the patients throughout their stay. The patient-focus unit radiographer will gain greater intrinsic rewards from the job due to the increased significance of their role in the successful treatment of individual patients.

3. *Team member*: being a team member of a multidisciplinary patient-focus unit team will broaden and enrich the radiographer's knowledge and understanding of other forms of care and their significance to the treatment of individual patients. As team members, they will build closer working relationships with other team members, therefore ensuring an increase in effective communication within the team.

4. *Reduced absenteeism and sickness*: the level of absenteeism and sickness may also reduce due to an increase in job satisfaction and team spirit.

Costs versus Savings

The high capital costs for the development of a patient-focus inpatient radiographic unit can be offset by savings on staff time. Table 5.1 demonstrates the flow of activities and the staff needed when the central department of one pilot site is used to obtain routine chest radiographs on medical inpatients. Table 5.2 illustrates the same process when a satellite patient-focus radiology unit is used at the same pilot site and when the patient-focus unit radiographer is involved in more team tasks. There are clearly process time and staff time savings to be made through utilization of a satellite patient-focus radiology unit.

Table 5.1   Chest radiographs in a central department

Step No.	Activity	Staff member responsible	Time taken* (s)
1	Complete request form	Doctor	90
2	Leave form with ward clerk	Doctor	15
3	Take request form to radiology department	Ward clerk	180
4	Hand in request form to radiology department	Ward clerk	30
5	Return to ward	Ward clerk	180
6	Sort requests	Radiology co-ordinator	30
7	Monitor and schedule X-ray slot	Radiology co-ordinator	180
8	Check patient availability	Radiology co-ordinator	180
9	Request inpatient slot	Radiology co-ordinator	30
10	Dispatch porter	Radiology co-ordinator	60
11	Travel to ward with chair	Porter	420
12	Retrieve X-rays from notes trolley	Ward clerk	90
13	Locate and verify patient	Porter and nurse	90
14	Move patient from bed	Porter and nurse	240
15	Transport to X-ray	Porter	420
16	Hand in films	Porter	30
17	Check details	X-ray receptionist	120
18	Enter data	X-ray receptionist	150
19	Put request form in designated slot	X-ray receptionist	15
20	Take request form to designated X-ray room	Radiology co-ordinator	60
21	Travel to patient waiting area	Radiographer	30
22	Identify patient	Radiographer	60
23	Take patient to designated X-ray room	Radiographer	60

Table 5.1   Continued

Step No.	Activity	Staff member responsible	Time taken* (s)
24	Put ID in chest changer	Radiographer	15
25	Position patient	Radiographer	180
26	Set machine	Radiographer	120
27	Take X-ray	Radiographer	15
28	Reseat patient	Radiographer	60
29	Auto film processing	Radiographer	90
30	Check X-ray quality	Radiographer	120
31	Number film and detail packet	Radiographer	90
32	Countersign request form	Radiographer	15
33	Put films out for transport to X-ray sorting room	Radiographer	30
34	Post patient's name as ready to return to ward	Radiographer	120
35	Identify patient for return to ward	Porter	60
36	Return patient to ward	Porter	420
37	Move patient into bed	Porter or nurse	240
38	Return to radiology department	Porter	420
39	Take films and request forms to be reported to sorting room	Porter	60
40	Marry up request forms and films	Filing clerk	150
41	Sort films by date	Filing clerk	30
42	Sort films by request	Filing clerk	30
43	Place into patient slot for reporting	Filing clerk	15
44	Collect films for reporting	Filing clerk or secretary	30
45	Read films	Radiologist	240
46	Dictate report	Radiologist	90
47	Type report and sort copies	Secretary	240
48	Validate report	Radiologist	60
49	Place packet in ward slot for collection	Secretary	15
50	Take packet to ward	Porter	60
51	Refile packet in notes trolley	Ward clerk	120
52	Retrieve packet from trolley and find latest films	Doctor	120
53	Read films	Doctor	240
54	Refile films on ward	Doctor or ward clerk	90
	Total		6345

*Times stated are averages and apply per patient when several patients' films are handled simultaneously.

Table 5.2   Chest radiographs in a patient-focus unit

Step No.	Activity	Staff member responsible	Time taken* (s)
1	Complete request form	Doctor	90
2	Drop off request form at satellite radiology facility	Doctor	30
3	Sort requests	Radiographer	30
4	Check patient availability	Radiographer	180
5	Travel to patient's bed with chair	Radiographer	60
6	Retrieve X-rays from notes trolley	Radiographer	90
7	Locate and verify patient	Radiographer and nurse	30
8	Move patient from bed	Radiographer and nurse	240
9	Transport to X-ray room	Radiographer	60
10	Enter data	Radiographer	150
11	Position patient	Radiographer	180
12	Set machine	Radiographer	120
13	Take X-ray	Radiographer	15
14	Reseat patient	Radiographer	60
15	Auto film processing	Radiographer	90
16	Naming of film	Radiographer	15
17	Check X-ray quality	Radiographer	120
18	Number film and detail packet	Radiographer	90
19	Countersign request form	Radiographer	15
20	Replace packet by patient	Radiographer	15
21	Return patient to patient's bed	Radiographer	60
22	Move patient into bed	Radiographer	240
23	Refile films in notes trolley	Radiographer	90
24	Return to radiology unit	Radiographer	60
25	Retrieve packet from trolley and find latest films	Doctor	120
26	Read films	Doctor	240
27	Refile films in notes trolley	Doctor	90
28	Collect films to be reported from notes trolley	Radiographer	60
29	Marry up request forms and films	Radiographer	120
30	Sort films by date	Radiographer	30
31	Sort films by request	Radiographer	30
32	Take films for reporting in central department	Radiographer	420
33	Return to ward area	Radiographer	420
34	Collect films for reporting	Secretary	30
35	Read films	Radiologist	240
36	Dictate report	Radiologist	90
37	Type report and sort copies	Secretary	240

Table 5.2   Continued

Step No.	Activity	Staff member responsible	Time taken* (s)
38	Validate report	Radiologist	60
39	Place packet in ward slot for collection	Secretary	15
40	Go to department to collect films	Radiographer	420
41	Collect reported films and return to ward area	Radiographer	60
42	Refile packet in notes trolley	Radiographer	90
	Total		4905

*Times stated are averages and apply per patient when several patients' films are handled simultaneously.

Arguably, it may also be considered wasteful and costly for highly trained radiographers to carry out transport and clerical duties. On-line, computer ordering of tests and retrieval of radiology reports and, ultimately, X-ray images, presently developed within certain UK hospitals, eliminate some of the process steps demonstrated in Table 5.1 and so speed up the process in centralized departments.

Costs and savings, if any, will differ from one patient-focus unit to another. The following factors should be considered when evaluating the financial and operational viability of developing a new satellite patient-focus radiology unit:

1. The number of patients to be x-rayed within the satellite patient-focus radiology unit.
2. Unit hours of work, for example, 24 hours per day, 365 days per year, bank holidays?
3. Patient type to be examined in the unit, for example, orthopaedic, surgical or medical patients.
4. Staffing levels and grade of patient-focus radiographer.
5. Unit overheads.
6. Geographical siting of the unit.
7. Existing information and imaging systems (on-line test ordering and report retrieval).
8. Amount of development funds available for purchase of equipment.
9. Suitability of patient-focus unit site for radiation protection, drainage of chemicals, ventilation and other technical requirements associated with radiography.

CONCLUSION

In conclusion, the development of an inpatient patient-focus radiology unit is a costly exercise which can create great benefits to patients, patient-focus unit staff and the central radiology department. Unfortunately, in an overstretched NHS economic climate, the benefits of patient-focused care may be overlooked and deemed non-cost-effective if all resources are not maximized. Time savings made through reducing the number of process steps and efficient use of staff time savings would not be recognized if staff time was not redeployed effectively. The multiskilling of staff could enhance jobs and increase the motivation of the workforce, if a careful and sensitive approach is taken when developing cross-boundary professional training. Adherence to, and observation of, statutory directives and regulations is crucial in ensuring safe professional practice.

The on-going development of further patient-focus radiology units heralds the necessity for specific patient-focus guidelines. These should include the following:

1. Professional governance should remain with the central radiology department.
2. Satellite units should participate fully in the internal and external quality-assurance programme advocated by the central radiology department.
3. The satellite radiology unit staff undertaking radiography must be state-registered radiographers.
4. Written protocols should be provided by the radiology department management and with the clinical advice of radiologists.
5. Non-radiographic staff carrying out support procedures should be trained and supervised by state-registered radiographers and should carry out duties within the protocols agreed by the central department.
6. Multidisciplinary skills required by state-registered radiographers should be underpinned by training based on strict systems of work.
7. Health and safety and radiation protection issues should be co-ordinated and controlled according to the central radiology department's procedures.

References

Black, A., Garside, P. (1994) Root and branch. In: Health Service Journal and Health Management Guide: Patient Focused Care. *Health Service Journal* (suppl.), 23 June: 1–2.

Carney, D. (1994) A Patient Focused Radiology Service – Benefits v Costs. Unpublished thesis May 1994.

Heyman, T., Culling, W. (1994) Medical unit X-ray facility. *British Medical Journal* **8 August**.

IBMS (1994) The IBMS view – patient focused services. *Biomedical Scientists*, **July:** 327.

Ionizing Radiations Regulations (1985) London: HMSO.

Ionizing Radiations (Protection of Persons Undergoing Medical Examinations or Treatment) Regulations (1988) London: HMSO.

Lathrop, J.P., Krouss, K.R., Shows, G.P. (1988) *Operational Restructuring – A Recipe for Success*. London: Booz-Allen and Hamilton.

Professions Supplementary to Medicine Act (1960) London: HMSO.

6

Radiographic Reporting in Diagnostic Imaging

Lyn McKay

Question: What is the difference between radiographers and radiologists?

Answer: Radiographers have always combed their own hair. Too cryptic for you? Then read on.

ROLE BOUNDARIES

In the early part of this century, hospitals employed radiographers to produce and comment upon x-ray images without medical supervision. This worked very well until the potential of these x-ray images was noted by the medical profession. Arguments about safety in the use and interpretation of X-rays were quickly put forward by the medical profession to try to justify an extension of medical control in this field (Larkin, 1983).

The arguments continued for a number of years, not only between the medical profession and the radiographers, but also between the radiographers themselves. Gender issues came to the fore, with male radiographers wishing to be viewed as technical experts, leaving the 'caring' side of the work to their female counterparts (Witz, 1992). This in-fighting played into the hands of the medical profession. The autonomy previously enjoyed by radiographers was removed and the emergence of the radiologist as a medical specialist ensued.

The terms 'radiographer' and 'radiologist' began to develop different meanings, although they did get confused. Radiologists went to great lengths to emphasize their difference from radiographers. Their aim was to establish radiology as a medical speciality. This was necessary to achieve the professionalization accorded to other medical specialities, that is, professional monopoly, autonomy and consultant status for radiologists.

In 1919, Hernaman-Johnson set out his ideas concerning the differences between radiographers and radiologists and gave advice to his fellow radiologists on how to tackle the problem:

> *Radiologists should organise and educate the various classes of lay helpers; to see that their status, remuneration and prospects are such as to make them contented; and to educate the public as to why such people are at one and the same invaluable as helpers, and extraordinarily dangerous when they seek to practise independently.*
>
> *(Hernaman-Johnson, 1919: 181)*

The role boundaries between radiographers and radiologists were thus created.

The distinction between the two occupations was exacerbated by their socialization into medical society, and later the health service, as the radiologists were seen as a 'true' professional group but radiographers were viewed as a 'semi' or 'para' professional group (Etzioni, 1969). These different strategies of socialization resulted in different consequences for each group, with the radiologists gaining control over the work situation and occupational sovereignty over radiographers (Turner, 1987).

The radiographer of later years has also been subjected to similar subordination, being viewed as a medical photographer, a 'button-pusher', even a hand-maiden to the radiologist, but not a professional with independence and autonomy (Larkin, 1983).

HAVE ROLES CHANGED?

With the recent moves towards self-governing trust hospitals and the consequential scrutiny of finances, hospital managers are under pressure to demonstrate effective use of the resources they have available to them. Reprofiling exercises are taking place to examine the quality of patient care balanced against cost-effective use of staff and, in this climate of change within the National Health Service (NHS), the concept of role expansion is gathering increasing interest.

Radiographers and radiologists each have an established role within an imaging department, but the previously rigid boundaries appear to be wavering. Radiographers trained in ultrasound theory and technique have infiltrated the radiological area of obstetric scanning. Indeed, in most parts of the country they are providing the whole of this service to the patient. They are also taking a broad role in general abdominal scanning. In some departments, radiographers are being taught the intricacies of barium enema examinations, an examination willingly relinquished by some radiologists. However, the field of imaging reporting seems to be a no-go area, with the radiologists hanging on to it as if their lives depended upon it.

Why should this be so? Is it because radiologists enjoy reporting so much, or is it because without the field of reporting their position of power may be called into question?

Some Facts

Radiologists have been expanding their own roles into interventional radiology and, with rapid advances in technology, this field grows ever wider. As the number of radiologists is not infinite, some areas of their work have, of necessity, received less attention. One of these areas is reporting. This has often resulted in reports not being produced in time, or at all, to influence the management of the patient. It has also been suggested that, even if a report is timely, accurate and well expressed, it may not be read, as some experienced specialist clinicians have little to learn in their field and do not require a report (Saxton, 1992). Saxton felt, therefore, that it was important that both radiologists and clinicians should co-operate to ensure that reports are noted and valued and take their place in the management of the patient.

Locally agreed guidelines and monitoring of incoming x-ray requests have had only a limited effect on reducing the reporting workload. In 1990, Fielding suggested that it should be possible to improve accident and emergency radiology significantly if the associated problems were defined and solutions were then constructed. He felt that one of the major problems was the status of the casualty officer. As casualty officers are usually junior doctors with little or no experience, they often made unnecessary requests and were then unable to interpret the images produced. A notable finding was that some radiologists regarded reporting as a chore. Fielding thought that, to combat both these problems, a radiographer abnormality-reporting system, commonly known as the 'red dot' system, should be introduced. This would help the inexperienced doctors and would take away some of the pressure associated with producing x-ray reports. His view was that the system used the experience of radiographers, but it 'rightly' stopped short of the contentious issue of making reports which he felt should remain the province of the radiologist. The red dot system has, indeed, proved to be very successful and was in use several years before Fielding's article. However, even this system of work is no longer sufficient.

In a study by Rose and Gallivan (1991) concerned with plain-film reporting in the UK, only 16% of the radiologists questioned believed that all examinations are reported. Often it is patients presenting from accident and emergency departments who are least well served in the majority of hospitals. The time has come for the role expansion of radiographers to be taken a step further, by developing their radiographic practices to enable them to provide written radiographic reports.

Radiographers are ideally placed to accept this particular development, as they have the necessary experience of pattern recognition, anatomy and pathology on which to build their image-interpretation skills. After radiographers have received essential, appropriate and systematic training, radiographic reports could be generated immediately following radiographic examinations. This would complement radiological reporting, improve the service to patients, and help reduce errors in patient management.

A TRAINING PROGRAMME FOR RADIOGRAPHERS

In support of this philosophy, staff at a hospital in the south of England, in conjunction with their local university's radiographic education unit, have produced a workplace-based education and training programme designed specifically to equip radiographers with the relevant and necessary knowledge to enable them to provide written radiographic reports. Initially this is to be for accident and emergency patients, but eventually patients from general practitioners would also receive a written radiographic report. This programme differs from the one offered through a northern hospital, as that is a pilot course for four radiographers only (Quick, 1993) and the training is taking place in a mainly academic atmosphere. The course offered at the southern site is on a larger scale. It aims to train all the radiographers in the hospital to carry out reporting in radiography, and is arranged so that the training takes place almost entirely in the diagnostic imaging department. The programme was originally developed as five modules of study. However, because of reservations outlined by radiology representatives during validation, only three of the modules were approved; approval of the modules relating to radiographic reporting of the abdomen and the thorax was deferred until further exploratory work had been conducted. Hence the programme structure now consists of three modules of postgraduate level, workplace-based study.

Module 1 provides the core elements required to develop further the skills related to radiographic reporting that radiographers already possess, as well as ethical and legal constraints to practice. Modules 2 and 3 concentrate on radiographic reporting of specific areas of the body, namely the appendicular skeleton and the axial skeleton. Each of these modules contains the necessary aspects of anatomy and physiology, pathology, pattern recognition, management of the patient and clinical reporting. At the end of the programme, if the radiographers have attained the required standards, a postgraduate certificate will be awarded. Eventually, once validation of the two remaining modules has been achieved, a postgraduate diploma will be available.

The workplace-based learning methods, together with academic tutor support, are relatively unexplored in radiography education. Research is to be undertaken to evaluate these innovative teaching and learning strategies. In addition, the impact of the course as a whole is to be evaluated rigorously.

RADIOGRAPHIC REPORTING – WHO GAINS?

Radiographers will gain by developing their abilities in pattern recognition and image analysis, by expanding the depth of their knowledge in anatomy and pathology, by playing a major role in the management of patients, and by receiving a postgraduate certificate in recognition of their efforts.

The hospital trust gains as it will be able to offer a high quality radiographic image reporting service to the accident and emergency department.

Patients gain as the reports offered by the radiographers will enhance the quality of care. Radiographic reports will be produced immediately following radiographic examinations throughout the full 24-hour, seven-day week cycle for which the accident and emergency department operates.

DO RADIOLOGISTS GAIN?

The programme has been developed to enable radiographers to fill a gap in the field of image reporting which exists in most hospitals. This should be a collaborative venture between radiographers and radiologists and not a game of role conflicts. A problem exists and this expansion of the role of the radiographer is an answer to that problem. Whether it will be viewed in this way remains to be seen. An article by Saxton (1992) which discussed the problem of too much work and too few radiologists suggested that radiographers, after relevant training, would be capable of providing reports on accident and emergency images. However, Saxton's article attracted a torrent of replies from radiologists in all parts of the country who were opposed to the idea. Interestingly, Saxton did feel that his article should have a health warning issued with it.

Whether radiologists like it or not, change and expansion in roles is a feature of today's professional. This is in tune with the reforms of the health service and with managers who are looking at the resources they have and the best ways in which to use them.

The traditional role of the radiographer is that of a producer of x-ray images. The traditional role of the radiologist is that of reporter of X-ray images. There is a need for these traditional roles to be disbanded and reformed as an amalgam. Radiographers should expand their role into image reporting. Radiologists should share this aspect of their work, so enabling their own role expansion into other fields. However, experience suggests that radiologists will feel that infringement of their role has taken place.

MANAGEMENT OF CHANGE

For both the radiographic and the radiological professions to be able to change, a radical remodelling in their socialization processes is required. In practice there is little encouragement for interprofessional collaboration within each profession's education and training programmes. The pity is that undergraduate education is the time and place to capture people's imaginations, when students begin to formulate, refine and adopt the values of their chosen professions. If an interprofessional trend is followed, this will remain with students past graduation (Castro, 1987). A natural progression of this would be for all health-care professionals to undergo a common foundation course in which they might learn about each other before they enter the world of the health service proper, where role boundaries create role conflict. If radiographers and radiologists could develop new ways of collaborating and sharing responsibilities, role expansion of radiographers into image reporting could become as successful as the red dot system. The determining factor should be what is best for the patient. If this means a readjustment of role expectations and a pooling of the knowledge and information of the two groups, then so be it.

EPILOGUE

Have you realised the meaning of the cryptic question and answer at the beginning of this article? No?

> *The radiographer should ensure the radiologist's hair is in place before he goes to face his public.*
>
> *(Lancet, 1952; in Larkin, 1983)*

Well, have radiographers' and radiologists' roles changed or not?

References

Castro, R.M. (1987) Preservice courses for interprofessional practice. *Theory into Practice* **26:** 103–109.

Etzioni, A. (1969) *The Semi-professions and their Organisations*. London: Collier Macmillan.

Fielding, J.A. (1990) Improving accident and emergency radiology. *Clinical Radiology* **41:** 149–151.

Hernaman-Johnson, F. (1919) The place of the radiologist and his kindred in the world of medicine. *Archives of Radiology and Electrotherapy* **24:** 181–187.

Larkin, G (1983) *Occupational Monopoly and Modern Medicine*. London: Tavistock.

Quick, J. (1993) Radiographers to interpret films. *Radiography Today* **59:** 1.

Rose, J.F., Gallivan, S. (1991) Plain film reporting in the UK. *Clinical Radiology* **44:** 192–194.

Saxton, H. (1992) Should radiologists report on every film? *Clinical Radiology* **45:** 1–3.

Turner, B.S. (1987) *Medical Power and Social Knowledge*. London: Sage.

Witz, A. (1992) *Professions and Patriarchy*. London: Routledge.

7

Developing Quality Standards in Radiography

David Dewitt

WHY SET STANDARDS?

Does the department in which you practise perform to high standards? Does the department produce high quality work?

If the answer to either of the above questions was 'yes', can it be proven? What criteria can be used to enable the standard of work in one department to be compared with that in any other?

Radiography departments have few agreed detailed performance specifications, though the College of Radiographers document *Guidelines for Provision of Acceptable Minimum Professional Standards of Care to be Specified in Contracts for Diagnostic Imaging and Interventional Services and Radiotherapy Services* does state many of the areas that a quality specification should cover.

Many National Health Service (NHS) Trusts, in a drive for greater efficiency within their organizations, are employing management consultancy firms to examine the operation of radiology and other services. Without clear objective quality standards, cost and productivity become the main criteria for examining a department's performance.

Productivity, cost and quality are all related issues and changing one of them can affect the other two. Working on the premise that quality issues must be included in the assessment of a department, how the relevant information is to be obtained needs to be determined.

PRODUCTIVITY

This is relatively staightforward information to obtain. Most radiology administration computer systems will quantify and analyse the work of a department.

COST

The true cost is difficult to assess. An imaging department has an annual budget for expenditure on aspects such as staff salaries, films, contrast media, and maintenance. However, the proportion of other hospital expenditure, for example heating, rates, administration, laundry and cleaning, which is apportioned to the department will vary, as individual finance departments may use different accounting procedures, and interpretations of the rules. This needs further discussion between radiology business managers and finance departments.

QUALITY

Subjectively, many staff would judge the work of a department using only two or three criteria, such as dose delivered per examination of any one type, quality control measures and final image appearances. These factors are totally inadequate as a means of assessing quality, and are more properly considered as matters of technical accuracy (accuracy being the closeness of an observed quantity to the defined or true quantity).

Hendra (1986) states that 'quality relates to the totality of features of a service that bear upon its ability to satisfy a given need'. Let us examine this statement in two parts. 'Totality of features' would include appointment systems, public areas, reception arrangements, film storage and retrieval systems, and many other issues such as technical proficiency of staff and reject rates. With regard to 'satisfy a given need', is the given need established? Do departments know what the consumers of the service (the customers) require or desire? How can this information be established? The obvious answer is ask the customers – but who are the customers? The answer may seem obvious, but different opinions exist.

Radiographers will often feel that the patients are the customers as the service is provided for their benefit. However, application of the British Standards Institute (BSI) quality-assurance approach to customer identification could suggest that the referring clinicians are the customers. Using this rationale, a customer is the person empowered to make decisions about whether to use a particular radiology service, an alternative diagnostic service, or the radiology service in another hospital. A clinician, who can refer to one or other specific x-ray department, or use an alternative service, such as endoscopy instead of a barium meal, is now the customer, and the patient becomes merely a passive component in a process. This matter will be returned to later.

The provision of a quality service requires the involvement and commitment of all members of staff of all disciplines and, therefore, the views of all the staff should be sought whilst identifying and quantifying the quality issues.

THE MISSION STATEMENT

At the start of this chapter, it was illustrated that, prior to writing any standards, the first stage is to identify and write down what exactly the department does – the services that are provided and for whom they are provided.

A policy statement, called a 'mission statement' or 'philosophy of care', should state concisely what the department's policy aims and beliefs are. A draft copy of this document should be prepared and circulated around the department for comments. This starts the process by which all members of staff can be consulted, because this statement must be agreed by everyone.

Having identified in broad terms the policy statement of the department, a more detailed analysis of the work is required. A method suggested by Hancock and Young (1992) is to set down the principal functions of the department. Try to restrict the number of these principal functions to no more than five or six in order to prevent the exercise from becoming unwieldy. It will also help to focus on the key areas of activity, one of which will be the service the department provides for patients. To achieve this limitation, concentrate on functions which each account for at least 10% of the department's time and effort. It is important when writing a principal function to indicate clearly what the service is and for whom it is provided. The principal functions will have identified who the customers of the department are – such as patients, referring clinicians, and purchasing health authorities.

The final step before standard setting is to set out the important components, these being all the activities necessary to carry out the principal function.

Who should Write the Standards?

Standards should be more than just a management control mechanism, they should constitute detailed descriptions of the functions and activities of the department. All staff have a role and need a commitment to achieving or improving the work standard. A group of mixed grades and disciplines and a customer representative, if possible, is ideal.

Writing the Standard

The *Oxford English Dictionary* defines a standard as 'an accepted example of something against which others are judged' or 'a measure to which others must conform'. In the present context, a useful definition is one used by Kitson et al. (1990): 'a professionally agreed level of performance'. Applying this to a radiography department, a standard is an objective performance specification against which the operation of the department can be measured.

The principal functions and important components will identify the subject areas for standard setting. A proforma is useful in preparing a standard; Figure 7.1 shows the modified form based on the Dynamic Standard Setting System used at Blackpool (Kitson et al., 1990). This proforma is filled in on the subject of patient waiting times to illustrate the information required.

The topic is the major area of the department's activity being analysed.

The customer group is the client group to whom this part of the service is delivered.

The subtopic is the detailed subject of the standard.

The standard statement states unambiguously the expectations of the standard. It is important not to use words like 'would' or 'should' or other terms which imply subjectivity, for example 'relevant' or 'appropriate'.

The three columns headed 'structure', 'process' and 'outcome' provide the means of determining whether a standard has been reached.

RADIOLOGY DEPARTMENT

STANDARD REF. NO:	1	DATE:	1 July 1994
TOPIC:	Clinical radiology service delivered to patients		
CUSTOMER GROUP:	Patients for non-contrast examinations	REVIEW DATE:	1 July 1995
SUBTOPIC:	Time patient (with appointment) waits till commencement of examination		
STANDARD STATEMENT:	ALL PATIENTS WITH APPOINTMENTS HAVE THEIR EXAMINATIONS STARTED WITHIN 30 MINUTES OF THEIR APPOINTMENT TIME		

STRUCTURE	PROCESS	OUTCOME
	This is achieved by:	All patients have their examinations started within 30 min
Office Manager provides: Staff time Appointment diary Film identification chits Receptionist	All preparatory clerical work is completed prior to the patient's arrival. Patient is asked to wait in waiting room	of their appointment time
Linen Manager must provide sufficient gowns	Patient is escorted to a cubicle, asked to undress, and put on a clean gown.	
A protocol for informing staff of patient attendance is in place	Receptionist notifies radiographer of the patient's attendance in the agreed manner	
Superintendent Radiographer provides: Imaging room/equipment Radiographers Consumables	An imaging room suitable for the task is available. A radiographer is available. Consumables are available	

Figure 7.1   Standard proforma.

1. *The Structure*: the people responsible, the local protocols and working practices which must exist to allow the process to occur.
2. *The Process:* the activities within the department which must occur to ensure an outcome.
3. *The Outcome*: the result(s) that must be achieved to ensure the standard is complied with.

Audit

Standard setting lays out what should happen, whereas audit measures how often, or whether it does. An example of an audit proforma is shown in Figure 7.2; again this is a modified form based on the Dynamic Standard Setting System.

The proforma shows that an audit merely involves converting every statement in the standard into a question. For example, the statement 'the office manger will ...' converts to 'did the office manager ...?'. Audit

RADIOLOGY DEPARTMENT

STANDARD REF. NO:	1
TOPIC	Clinical radiology service delivered to patients
CUSTOMER GROUP:	Patients for non-contrast examinations
SUBTOPIC:	Time patient (with appointment) waits till commencement of examination
STANDARD STATEMENT:	ALL PATIENTS WITH APPOINTMENTS HAVE THEIR EXAMINATIONS STARTED WITHIN 30 MINUTES OF THEIR APPOINTMENT TIME

Audit date: _____ Standard audited by: _____

Source of information	Criteria	Yes	No	Does not apply
Observe/documentation	Was all preparatory clerical work completed prior to the patient's arrival?			
Observe	Was patient escorted to a cubicle, asked to undress and put on a clean gown?			
Observe/enquire	Was an imaging room suitable for the task available?			
Observe/enquire	Was a radiographer available?			
Observe/enquire	Were consumables available?			
Enquire Documentation Documentation Observe	Did the office manager provide: Staff time? Appointment diary? Film identification chits? Receptionist?			
Observe	Were sufficient gowns available?			
Observe	Was radiographer notified of patient's arrival in agreed manner?			
Enquire Enquire Enquire	Did Superintendent Radiographer provide: Imaging room? Radiographer? Consumables?			
Enquire	Was a protocol for informing staff of patient's attendance in place?			
Observe	Did the patient's examination start within 30 min of their appointment time?			

Figure 7.2   Audit proforma.

should be carried out by someone not involved in writing the standard and, if possible, by someone external to the department. To facilitate external audit, standards and audits should be clear and avoid jargon. Some standards, for example, standards on technical excellence, will need a person of specific expertise to validate statements; perhaps a neighbouring department could supply radiographers for this task.

The frequency of audit of each standard is a matter for local decision, but once a year should be a minimum. The caseload looked at by each audit is again a matter for a local decision. The audit should include a sufficient number of cases for it to be representative.

Scoring the audit is a matter of determining how many things *did* happen compared with how many things *should* have happened, and expressing this as a percentage.

Timetable and Review

The process of standard setting requires a timetable to ensure that standards are set and audited in a planned and systematic manner. Planning should encompass at least 6 and probably the next 12 months.

Departmental functions, workload, and staff changes produce a need to review standards. Therefore, each standard is dated (Figure 7.1) and states the expected review date.

An annual review is probably sufficient, but major change may require an earlier review.

Validation of Standards and Consultation with Customer Groups

At the beginning of this chapter, quality was related to 'satisfying a given need'. One way of establishing whether the standards achieve this aim is to ask the customers. Patient satisfaction questionnaires and user ward/department questionnaires should be used routinely to establish if the department's service is perceived to be of high quality by its customers. The results of these surveys should be fed back into the standards setting process where appropriate.

CONCLUSION

Asking the staff of an imaging department about 'standards' and 'quality' is not always the best method of establishing the performance of a department. Written standards state the objective performance standards that a department strives to achieve, and audit shows how successful it is in achieving them.

All departments are different and, although certain objectives will be common, each department can use this exercise to demonstrate its own priorities.

Finally, departments should publish their standards and the audit results for their customers and demonstrate a commitment to quality which is clear for everyone to see.

References

College of Radiographers (1990) *Guidelines for Provision of Acceptable Minimum Professional Standards of Care to be Specified in Contracts for Diagnostic Imaging and Interventional Services and Radiotherapy Services.* London: The College of Radiographers.

Hancock C.P., Young, D. (1992) *A Practical Framework for Quality Evaluation.* North Kelsey, Lincs: Lake View Learning.

Hendra, I.R.F. (1986) A systematic approach to quality assurance in medical diagnostic imaging. *Institute of Physics Short Meetings Series No .2 'Quality Assurance in Medical Imaging',* 5 August 1986. London: Institute of Physics.

Kitson, A., Hyndman, S., Harvey, G. et al. (1990) *Quality Patient Care – The Dynamic Standard Setting System.* RCN Standards of Care Project. London: Royal College of Nursing.

8

Quality Accreditation – What Cost?

Stephen A. Evans

INTRODUCTION

In North America, some countries of Europe and in Australasia, accreditation is well established. The National Health Service (NHS), however, holds accreditation at arm's length, as though wary it might bite. The *Pocket Oxford Dictionary* (1984) defines 'accredit' as: 'gaining belief or influence'. To be accredited is to be 'officially recognized; generally accepted and believed'. What, therefore, concerns the NHS?

Healy (1988), writing on health-care quality-assurance terminology, gives the World Health Organization (WHO) description of accreditation: 'the process by which an agency or organization evaluates and recognizes a programme of study or institution as meeting predetermined standards'.

In 1988, King Edward's Hospital Fund for London (The King's Fund) reported upon various international accreditation programmes. Their research culminated in the King's Fund Organizational Audit, to which many NHS hospitals now voluntarily subscribe. This popular and effective organizational audit is potentially a precursor to NHS accreditation. The King's Fund (1988) states that:

Health care accreditation addresses issues of evaluating the quality of health services provided. It is the professional and national recognition reserved for facilities that provide high quality health care. This means that the particular health care facility has voluntarily sought to be measured against high professional standards and is in substantial compliance with them. It differs from both registration and licensing in that it is not a statutory but a voluntary system.

All accreditation systems share essentially the same elements (King's Fund, 1988):

1. An accreditation board constituted of representatives of professional and health-care organizations and in some countries, of government and consumer interests.
2. Comprehensive standards developed to reflect current practice, extensively reviewed by practitioners with expertise in the area.
3. Surveyors chosen and trained to apply the standards to a specific health-care service. This involves site visits by the surveyors, who make suggestions for improvement and recommend to the board whether or not to grant accreditation.

The King's Fund recommends that:

1. The system should be voluntary.
2. Surveys should be comprehensive in intent.
3. Survey teams should be multidisciplinary, based on the principle of peer review.
4. Surveying methods, approaches and standards should be stated openly, for public scrutiny and challenge.

Accreditation is thus a process of voluntary peer review, whereupon the organization is measured against standards that are subject to public and professional scrutiny.

In recent years, the NHS has improved its quality management, yet still there is no comprehensive system for comparing health-care quality throughout the UK. Variable systems and standards characterize the NHS. The Government White Paper *Working for Patients* (HM Government, 1989) fuelled interest in 'quality' as a negotiable *measure* of care by introducing the 'health market' and purchaser/provider split. The 1989 reforms were vague, however, about what 'quality' means and how it might be measured. The NHS is now driven by contracts written in terms of cost, volume and *quality*. Typically, the 'quality' content of current NHS contracts refers principally to maximum waiting times. The consequence of such a fixed approach is likely to be deterioration in many other aspects of quality delivery, unless these too are measurably specified and better reported. In this lies the reason for an accreditation system.

Through NHS contracting, purchasing organizations such as health authorities and general practice fund holders buy care for their populations. Purchasers encourage competition and should buy from the best provider, giving due regard to the needs and preferences of the people for whom they purchase. Thus is accreditation needed? The answer lies in another question: Do purchasers have the resources, knowledge and *right* to specify and monitor the optimum provision of every clinical service? Such a specification would be complex. It could be produced, but by whom and for whom? A good contract maintains a delicate balance among three vital elements: volume, cost and quality. Each directly affects the other two. Cost and volume are definable and increasingly non-negotiable, but quality is ever more the essential variable. It is getting harder to determine and monitor – particularly as the competitive market environment takes hold.

If the purchaser specifies quality requirements, in whose terms are they written? The purchaser's own, or their professional or political masters? Should they be written in the patient's interests, or is that society's best interests? If the purchaser specifies standards for the process of delivery, can the purchaser also specify the outcome? But if the purchaser specifies outcome, what might be the costs of guaranteeing it? The familiar adage 'the operation was successful but the patient died' is a succinct statement of process and outcome. Does the purchaser specify the standards for the operation, or demand that the patient lives?

O'Leary and Schyve (1993) distinguish between standards and outcome in appealing to the Clinton Administration to consider how care will be measured in a reformed US health-care system:

> Standards are simply statements of performance expectations that, if followed, should lead to good outcomes. The two types of measurement complement each other. Outcomes are measures of past performance; compliance with relevant standards is a predictor of future good performance. Past outcomes are predictors of future outcomes only if the processes that produced them are stable. Good outcomes can be obtained only if the processes involved are implemented in accordance with current state-of-the-art knowledge – as reflected in standards.

O'Leary and Schyve fear the US system will become outcomes obsessed and lose interest in the standard-setting process which ensures that consistent state-of-the-art procedure is followed. In so doing, outcomes may improve, but care may become more variable, expensive and complex in order to assure the outcome and thus, as costs inevitably rise, health care becomes less accessible.

So there is a dilemma. It is possible to specify process and/or outcome through contracting. But in so doing, the purchaser may develop a conflicting specification that fails to meet the needs of those the purchaser represents (politician and patient) and, above all, limits the real objective – the best standards applied to bring about the optimum outcome with value for money. I argue here that purchasers should limit their contractual demands for a 'quality' service to requiring provider accreditation by a national body that effectively defines and evaluates standards of service delivery.

THE BASIS OF ACCREDITATION

Accreditation is a standards-based process of evaluation. In making standards for service measurable and reliable, consumer and purchaser requirements can be professionally served by the provider. This is accreditation's potential. Accreditation asks those providing services to volunteer to be judged by their peers against standards developed by both their peers and others with an interest in the organization and its services. Truly effective accreditation standards are measurable by those who buy care, deliverable by those who provide it and acceptable to those who receive care. The standards should comply with Maxwell's (1984) dimensions for the quality of health-care delivery, being efficient, effective, equitable, appropriate, acceptable and accessible to all.

US and Australian accreditation programmes have been criticized for being oriented towards process rather than outcome. They concentrate on the right documentation and correct procedure, without significant regard for the effect those elements have upon quality of care. For this reason, both countries' accrediting bodies are working with the medical profession to develop clinical-outcome indicators. These indicators will be fundamental to a truly comprehensive accreditation system. An NHS system should seek a balance between performance standards and outcome measures.

O'Connor and Wolff (1993) criticize the Australian accreditation process for its emphasis on structure without regard to outcome. They feel that accreditation should determine whether hospitals which meet the appropriate standards and, therefore, have the capability to deliver high-quality care, have done so. O'Connor and Wolff are concerned that the accreditation survey is treated cynically by staff who witness frantic activity leading up to a survey and then see the hospital fall back to 'normal' until the next survey is due. This may be prevented by engendering a desire amongst staff for continuous improvement. The key contribution to accreditation standards should be from staff themselves.

THE IMPACT OF ACCREDITATION

Accreditation is widely perceived to lack effective sanctions and rewards. A hospital may be unable to operate effectively without accreditation, but having achieved it there is little incentive for continuous and rigorous improvement. Dick Davidson, President of the American Hospitals Association, comments upon the need to strengthen voluntary accreditation and give teeth to the accrediting body. He is keen to 'increase public disclosure about hospital shortcomings' to support 'growing demand for clear, credible information about providers'. (Davidson, 1993). He understands that 'sceptics question the validity of pre-scheduled accreditation visits ... [because] when lapses are found there's little penalty'. Davidson says a 'more rigorous accreditation process will help US hospitals be more accountable to patients and payers' and he notes that the accrediting body 'is acknowledging that quality of care matters more than quantities of forms and paperwork'. Davidson looks forward to an accreditation system which 'will eventually make it easier to demonstrate and maintain high quality, to compare prices with quality and to identify and understand the trade-offs involved in various cost-control strategies'.

Accreditation puts quality of care at the centre, without losing sight of the need for efficiency and cost-effectiveness. When all NHS purchasers and providers negotiate contracts around standards determined by an independent accrediting body, the result should be nationally comparable, deliverable services, realistically resourced.

SO WHAT PRICE ACCREDITATION?

Accreditation by an independent organization is expensive. The US Joint Commission on the Accreditation of Health Care Organizations (JCAHO) has an annual budget in excess of $35 million. Providers pay for accreditation, and considerable expense is necessary to prepare for the survey. It could be argued that the money might otherwise buy health care. An opposing argument must be that a well-operated accreditation programme will promote efficient and effective care delivery and bring about better access to services.

Some fear that the price of accreditation is loss of professional freedom. Standard-based systems raise concerns about production-line techniques and constraining procedures. This echoes criticism of BS 5750: 1987 in the clinical environment. BS 5750: 1987 is a form of accreditation. Organizations with BS 5750: 1987 have demonstrated their ability to operate in a consistent and reliable manner. They document their activities and do not deviate from them without following an appropriate process to justify and test the change. BS 5750: 1987 is not concerned with the outcome of the activity, merely the process. Every widget may be faulty, but the British Standards Institution would expect to see the same fault consistently. That way rectification is straightforward. A different fault every time suggests disorganized and chaotic practice. This translates well to health care.

Standard setting for health-care accreditation requires input from professional staff involved in the care activity. A standard must be acceptable to staff required to exceed it in practice. Professional freedom is compromised only if the professionals fail to put sufficient commitment into developing, maintaining and owning the standards. The key seems to be to find the motivating factor that builds and sustains such commitment.

Accreditation should serve purchasers, consumers and providers equally. Achieving this balance requires significant changes in purchasing strategy, public perception and the manner of delivery. Providers may have to learn to do things differently. If this brings more and better care, more consistently and, more quickly, who can oppose the change? The greatest opposition will come from the professionals – unless they are involved in developing the standards to which they will work.

This raises the issue of who owns standards. Standard setting requires input from buyers, providers and users of a service. Which dominates? Bias towards a faction is apparent in all existing accreditation systems. Generally, the bias favours the payer – the government or the insurance company.

Independent NHS accreditation should complement the contracting system, precluding the need for extensive negotiation of quality parameters. Clinical staff often feel they are insufficiently involved in contracting. This is perhaps because contract negotiation is currently an exercise in meeting political and financial targets that have limited regard for service quality. Ultimately, quality of service is internally negotiated, and hence there are wide variations from provider to provider, and region to region. Accreditation may be the clinician's route into effective control of contracting.

Purchasers increasingly struggle to match public aspirations with political prerogative. An accreditation programme that brings together the public, professional, managerial and political players may focus the presently anarchic activities surrounding the purchasing of NHS health care.

WHAT MIGHT ACCREDITATION MEAN TO THE NHS?

Purchasers have difficulty in making robust comparisons of providers. Providers too, are unable to assess their relative performance. Advances are being made in cost comparisons using health-care related groups (HRGs). HRGs indicate the relative price efficiency of each provider offering clinical work requiring similar resources. Still missing from the formula is evidence of how closely care delivery matches current knowledge and the state of the clinical art. A national system of accreditation standards, developed by buyers, providers and users of care, might reassure purchasers and patients that their provider is cost-effective and meets the current quality criteria. The King's Fund suggests that common standards will promote development of a national framework for co-ordinated quality assurance and an active debate on the standard-setting exercise.

Accreditation identifies services that fall below minimum standards or fail to improve at an acceptable rate. It indicates services needing additional resource to match the best and reveals those that are over-resourced or no longer cost- or care-effective.

Providers volunteering for accreditation directly benefit in many ways. They can evaluate their services through peer review. Handled well, the accreditation survey can motivate staff to confront existing problems. Those participating in the King's Fund Organizational Audit know that the exercise is effective in generating a multidisciplinary approach, breaking down traditional barriers and encouraging a new approach to old issues.

Staff can demonstrate operational excellence and be involved in preparing the service for peer review leading to accreditation. After accreditation is gained, staff should be encouraged to deliver the continuing improvements necessary to exceed future standards. Such staff involvement requires that they consider all aspects of service delivery, from the political and purely financial standpoint to the patient's view. This is a challenge for managers.

Accreditation provides a positive message for health-care organizations to communicate to staff, patients, the media and purchasers. In a competitive system it helps attract new business and the best staff.

For the user of a health organization's services, accreditation offers independent and expert evaluation of good practice and quality of care. Patients, their carers and representatives have the opportunity to participate in standards development and the accreditation process.

CONCLUSION

Voluntary accreditation focuses the quality management of health care around the needs and wants of all those with an interest. Developed well, an NHS accreditation programme will pull together the disparate quality and contracting activities of a fragmented service. It will produce a singular approach nationwide, putting the quality spotlight on the patient. It will encourage value for money and incorporate the clinical view.

However, none of this will be achieved without readiness on the part of health professionals to accept that their services may change radically to meet the demands of an accreditation programme which genuinely serves all stakeholders in care.

References

British Standards Institution (1987) *BS 5750 British Standard Quality Systems*. Milton Keynes: British Standards Institution.

Davidson, D. (1993) JCAHO accreditation at the crossroads. *Hospitals and Health Networks* p 12.

Healy, S. (1988) Health care quality assurance terminology. *International Journal of Health Care Quality Assurance* 1: 20–32.

H.M. Government (1989) *Working for Patients* (White Paper). London: HMSO.

King Edward's Hospital Fund for London (1988) *Health Service Accreditation – an International Overview*. London: King's Fund Centre.

Maxwell, R.J. (1984) Quality assessment in health. *British Medical Journal* 288: 470–471.

O'Connor, P.T., Wolff, A.M. (1993) Preparation for hospital accreditation: an efficient and practical approach. *Australian Clinical Review* 13: 157–163.

O'Leary, D.S., Schyve, P.M. (1993) The role of accreditation in quality oversight and improvement under healthcare reform. *The Quality Letter*. Dec. 1993–Jan. 1994.
Pocket Oxford Dictionary, 7th edn. Oxford: Clarendon Press (1984).

Bibliography

Calman, K.C. (1992) Quality: a view from the centre. *Quality in Health Care* **1** (Suppl.): S28–S33.
Morgan, J., Everett, T. (1990) Introducing quality management in the NHS. *International Journal of Health Care Quality Assurance* **3:** 23–36.
Moss, F. (1992) Achieving quality in hospital practice. *Quality in Health Care* **1** (Suppl): S17–S19.
Randall, A. (1992) Hospitals get the quality treatment. *Financial Times* **6 March**.
Roberts, H. (1990) Ins and outcomes. *The Health Service Journal.* **1 Nov.:** 1653–1654.
Rutgers, M., Berkel, H. (1990) New concepts in health care: some preliminary ideas. *International Journal of Health Planning and Management* **3:** 221–226.

9

Dose Reduction in Diagnostic Imaging

Timothy Reynolds

INTRODUCTION

At a time when role extension in radiography is high on the agenda, it could be argued that there must be assurances that key aspects of current roles are not abdicated prior to agreeing new ones. In this respect the wider consideration of radiation dosimetry and the informed application of appropriate radiation protection measures are important. There is no room for complacency. Radiographers, because of the nature of their work, must be knowledgeable in the field of radiation protection. While radiographers might not claim expert status, they would assert that they know all that is required for practical purposes.

When questioning radiographers attending recent College of Radiographers legal issues seminars in Oxford, Glasgow, Manchester and London, it became clear that they believed the level of awareness within the profession in relation to radiation protection is greater than that of referring clinicians. This view was reinforced during similar questioning at radiation protection study days held throughout the West Midlands during 1993. At each of these seminars and study days radiographers indicated that, in their opinion, the courses for delivery of the 'Core of Knowledge' (Ionizing Radiations Regulations, 1988) were inadequate.

Inadequate 'Core of Knowledge' courses, although a cause for alarm, are not the concern of this chapter. Such inadequacies lend weight to the case for radiographers to act as 'gate keepers' and to filter out unneccesary radiographic examinations. For this to happen successfully, radiographers need to demonstrate a high level of knowledge and skill. This chapter examines the level of awareness of radiation protection demonstrated by radiographers. All qualifying courses in radiography include the essential elements of the 'Core of Knowledge', but how much of this is carried past the exit of the examination rooms?

It is likely that most radiographers employ practical radiation protection measures, for example, collimation and gonad protection, for the majority of the time. The term 'most' is used deliberately because even these basic requirements are not utilized by all radiographers. This assertion is based on personal observation made during visits to a number of x-ray departments seeking accreditation for student training. The observations cover a range of failures in radiation protection practice from that which was questionable to that which may be considered as a total disregard for regulations and local rules.

The important question is how widespread are these lapses?

THE EVIDENCE

In January 1991, *Which?* magazine published an article that was critical of radiation protection practices. The article was based on a number of interviews with patients who had undergone diagnostic x-ray procedures. The findings of the survey indicated, at best, a lack of awareness or, at worst, negligence. Some of the problems highlighted were:

1. Around 50% of patients were not questioned about previous x-ray examinations of the same part of the body.
2. Where patients were questioned, in more than two-thirds of cases it was not until the examination had taken place .
3. Almost 30% of patients of child-bearing age were not questioned about the possibility of being pregnant.

The College of Radiographers, in a press release in 1991, conceded that there was scope for dose reductions in diagnostic radiology, but added that for this to become reality adequate funds would have to be made available to replace obsolete equipment. If a national replacement programme for x-ray equipment were to be contemplated, a major part of the responsibility for dose reduction would be placed on the Department of Health as the holder of the purse strings. Acceptance of this standpoint would provide an easy option for radiographers and their managers. Dose monitoring and review of radiation protection and examination protocols could be deferred on the basis that efforts to reduce radiation doses were hindered by obsolete radiation-producing equipment. The merits of this argument are called into question by a study carried out by Calverd (1993). His results showed no correlation between the age of equipment and the radiation dose to the patient.

Criticism of the *Which?* report was directed justifiably at the method of investigation. The survey of a little more than 2000 subjects revealed that around 25% had undergone diagnostic x-ray procedures within the previous year. These patients were interviewed about their experiences regarding radiation protection measures and the article was based on the recollection of events which had taken place as much as 12 months previously.

The results are questionable because patients who are or who have been in a stressful situation are unlikely to have total recall of either practical measures which were applied or of conversations between themselves and the radiographers. This is particularly true following a delay of up to 12 months. Despite the flawed methodology it must be accepted that a number of the reported omissions will have taken place.

The number of accurately recorded incidents is not the critical factor. Whether 1% or 100% of the stated examples of inadequate professional practice or negligence took place, the figure should have been zero. Each of the faults recorded were in everyday, practical radiation protection measures – the area in which radiographers should perform well.

Radiographers physically directing ionizing radiations are required to be 'adequately trained'. This is defined in Statutory Instrument (SI) 778; that is the Ionizing Radiations Regulations (1988) or the POPUMET (Protection of Persons undergoing Medical Examinations or Treatment) Regulations. These regulations require that those physically directing ionizing radiations receive 'tuition leading to competence in radiation protection and appropriate instruction including practical experience in the diagnostic or therapeutic procedures to be used'.

The schedule of SI 778 sets out what is termed the 'Core of Knowledge', that is an outline of the knowledge that is required by those who are to act in the capacity of physically directing radiation doses. The term 'Core of Knowledge' is familiar to radiographers, but the contents less so. This assertion is, again, made on the basis of College of Radiographers legal issues seminars and West Midlands study days. The total number of radiographers attending these seminars and courses was in excess of 400. A small sample of the radiographer population maybe, but a sample which had demonstrated at least some awareness of the need to update their knowledge.

The requirement for a detailed knowledge of the nature of ionizing radiations and their effects does not end with the awarding of a diploma or a degree in radiography. The body of knowledge within this subject is changing constantly and there is both a legal and an ethical requirement for radiographers to update their knowledge continually.

Radiographers reading this chapter may be somewhat indignant that, effectively, their professionalism is being questioned. However, they should, first, consider the following questions:

1. Which carries the greater radiation weighting factor?
   (a) Gamma rays.
   (b) X-rays.
2. Which carries the greater tissue weighting factor?
   (a) Red bone marrow.
   (b) The colon.
3. Describe the following attenuation processes and their effect on the radiographic image:
   (a) Photoelectric effect.
   (b) Compton scatter.
4. Define the terms:
   (a) Deterministic.
   (b) Stochastic.

Those who cannot answer these questions do not fulfil the requirements of the first two requirements within the 'Core of Knowledge'.

It may be felt that consideration of such points is not of great importance in the day-to-day work of the radiographer when making practical decisions about the management of a patient's examination. However, in the process of seeking professional autonomy and equal status with other health-care professionals, the radiographer must be able to discuss and justify with their clinical colleagues the decisions they make.

The graphs shown in Figure 9.1 refer to deterministic and stochastic effects of ionizing radiation (Hughes, 1991), but which graph applies to

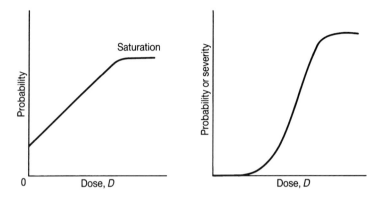

Figure 9.1   Probability – dose curves for deterministic and stochastic
effects of radiation (After Hughes, 1991).

which type of effect? The answer may be obvious but what do these
graphs mean in terms of the practical considerations for radiographers? Again, when discussing the advisability of undertaking a particular examination referring clinicians, assuming they take their
responsibilities seriously, may want to know:

1. Whether the radiation damage will be repaired.
2. Whether the fact that the patient has had a similar examination
   will increase the risk by a factor of 2.

The latter, of course, depends on the risk response being linear and the
dose accumulation being arithmetic. The answers to both questions differ, depending on the type of effect.

Perhaps more important for the radiographer is the question of the
relationship between dose rate and the deterministic and stochastic
effects of ionizing radiation. For one type of effect the severity depends
on dose and dose rate, while in the other it is independent of dose rate.
How many radiographers can say which statement refers to which
effect?

In 1986, the National Radiological Protection Board (NRPB) published a document detailing the results of a dosimetry survey undertaken at 20 UK hospitals (Shrimpton et al., 1986). Doses were recorded
for a range of common examinations. The survey demonstrated, as suggested subsequently in the *Which?* article, that there is considerable
variation in the radiation doses received by patients at different hospitals. Extracts from the survey are shown in Table 9.1.

At the time of the dosimetry survey, many departments were not

Table 9.1 Some results of the National Radiological Protection Board Dosimetry Survey

	Entrance surface dose (mGy)	
	Minimum	Maximum
Lumbar spine		
Anteroposterior	0.83	59.1
Lateral	2.38	108.0
Sacroiliac joints	7.40	131.0
Abdomen		
Anteroposterior	0.71	62.4
Skull		
Anteroposterior	0.73	13.9
Lateral	0.36	9.09

using high-speed recording systems. It could be assumed that these departments would be those at the upper end of the dose range. However, this should no longer be the case.

The National Dosimetry Protocol, jointly published in 1992 by the NRPB, the Institute of Physical Sciences in Medicine and the College of Radiographers, was designed to assess the current levels of radiation dose being delivered. Early results from the protocol indicate that doses are being reduced. But, do all radiographers know how the doses delivered currently in the departments in which they work compare with those published in 1986?

The answer should be 'Yes' as the 'Core of Knowledge' requires that those physically directing ionizing radiations are aware of the range of doses for examinations carried out, the factors affecting dose, and the methods of dose measurement. This legal requirement cannot be devolved to a few individuals with enthusiasm and interest.

This legal requirement was further supported in the Guidance Notes for the Protection of Persons Against Ionizing Radiations Arising from Medical or Dental Use (NRPB, 1988). Paragraph 2.12 of this document effectively makes provision for those with no access to dose-measuring devices by advising that, following an examination, details relevant to the estimation of radiation dose should be recorded.

All radiographers should be aware of the radiation dose they are likely to be delivering every time they carry out an examination. Experience of the numerous study days and seminars suggests that few could make such a claim. The lack of awareness of radiation protection matters is alarming, particularly given the increased publicity about radiation during the past 2–3 years. Not only have there been articles such as that in *Which?*, but also items in the national press and on the radio. Much of this publicity has been as a result of the publication in 1990 of ICRP(60). This document, from the International Commission for Radiation Protection, detailed factors which have led to a three-fold increase in risk estimates due to exposure to ionizing radiation. The need, therefore, for radiographers to take an interest in and to take appropriate radiation-dose minimizing actions becomes ever more important.

What might be the result if radiographers fail to carry out their role in relation to radiation protection? Notwithstanding the ethical considerations of providing the best possible care for patients in their charge, radiographers who do not comply with the requirements of the 1985 and 1988 ionizing radiations legislation run the risk of prosecution. The purpose of this chapter is not to alarm, but there will always be circumstances in which accidental exposures and overdoses take place. When this happens, if the incident is properly dealt with and investigated, no one is likely to end up in a court of law, although if a single radiographer is involved in a number of such incidents questions must be asked.

The most serious incidents, and hence those more likely to result in legal action or action by the professional and state registration bodies, are those involving wilful negligence. Radiographers are professional, caring people who would not do anything willingly that was likely to harm either their patients or their own professional future. Wilful negligence is, therefore, unusual and extremely rare.

PRACTICE SITUATIONS

How, then, do the comments made here relate to the practice of the majority of radiographers who work with steady and reliable colleagues? Are the following scenes familiar?

A radiographer enters the staff room and makes coffee. Turning to the room, the radiographer says:

'Exposures in Room 2 are a bit down, you need to go up by about 5 kVp'.

or

'The diaphragms in Room 1 are a bit out when using a horizontal beam'.

These are not unusual conversations and, if all in the coffee room then go about their normal business, no 'major' overdoses are likely to occur. But, it must be remembered that not all harmful effects are dose-dependent, and every radiographer who uses Rooms 1 and 2 that day will have acted with wilful negligence and will have contravened both the 1985 and the 1988 Ionizing Radiations Regulations. This claim is possible because, without proper testing of the faulty equipment, it cannot be known whether the faults highlighted during the coffee break conversation are constant. The performance of the equipment cannot, therefore, be guaranteed.

In addition, altering exposure factors or field of radiation to compensate for the problems may, or may not, result in the production of a diagnostic image. If it does not and a repeat projection is required, the radiation dose to the patient will have doubled. Half of that dose will be totally unjustifiable. In such circumstances it would be difficult to build a defence to show that due diligence had been applied and all precautions had been taken to ensure that the dose complied with the ALARP (as low as reasonably practicable) principle – a patient will have been exposed to ionizing radiation on equipment known to be faulty.

TRAINING

A similar situation may be portrayed in relation to 'adequate training', as laid down in the Ionizing Radiations Regulations 1988. 'Adequate training' does not simply mean instruction on radiation protection topics during the qualifying period. It also covers training on new equipment after qualifying.

Question: A radiographer is required to work on equipment that has been installed recently. A patient overdose occurs because the operator is not sure how each aspect of the equipment works. What is the defence?

Answer: There is none.

Employing authorities have an obligation to ensure that those physically directing ionizing radiation are adequately trained and, if they fail in this duty, they will not be safe from action. This responsibility, however, is no greater than that of the operators themselves to ensure that they are competent on that new piece of equipment.

RADIATION-DOSE REDUCTION STRATEGIES

Published figures from the NRPB (1989) show that 15% of the radiation dose to the UK population is from manmade sources. Of this, 90%, or up to 20000 man-sieverts, arises from medical uses. It has been suggested by the NRPB and the Royal College of Radiologists (1990) that a reduction in total UK radiation dose of approximately 50% is possible without detriment to patient care. This is a significant figure, and everyone involved in work with ionizing radiation must play their part to achieve this goal.

A major factor in possible dose-reduction strategies is quality-assurance systems. Calverd (1993) addressed this subject. From measurements made in a number of departments, he was able to demonstrate considerable dose reductions following the introduction of processor quality-assurance alone. Other quality-assurance factors then brought yet greater reductions in radiation dose. The College of Radiographers (1992) guidelines on the introduction of quality-assurance programmes also link quality assurance and radiation dose inextricably: 'monitoring radiation dose is central to a quality assurance programme'.

Far too often the question of quality is the remit of one or two radiographers within a department who show a particular interest in the subject. But, quality assurance is not only desirable, it is a legal requirement specified within the 'Core of Knowledge' and, hence, all radiographers should involve themselves in the quality question and quality-assurance procedures.

A further factor in reducing radiation dose to the population is the requirement for exposures to ionizing radiations to be justified in all cases. There are many examples of unjustified requests for X-ray examinations. These include inappropriate requests such that the examination requested will not best demonstrate the suspected pathology, and requests for examinations where retrieval of previous films would have removed the need for the current examination. Figures, again from the NRPB and the Royal College of Radiologists (1990), show that approximately 20% of the total UK radiation dose falls into this category of unjustified examination requests.

The NRPB suggest that this unnecessary dose could account for between 100 and 250 of the 160000 cancer deaths each year, that is between 0.06% and 0.16% of all cancer deaths. (Also reported in the national press, Hawkes (1991).) This is not a large percentage, but what percentage is acceptable in terms of unnecessary deaths due to unnecessary radiation? Lives saved are, surely, worthwhile.

RADIOGRAPHERS' ROLE

What then, is the role of the radiographer in minimizing the radiation dose to the population? Requests for radiological examinations are not usually seen by a radiologist prior to those examinations taking place, and many of the resulting radiographs may not be reported prior to treatment being initiated or changed. Who, then, provides the expert advice to the referring clinician as to the appropriateness of the X-ray request? It must be the radiographer acting as the gate keeper of the system.

There is no compulsion on the part of the radiographer to complete an examination simply because it has been requested by a medical practitioner. Radiographers can, and must, refuse to carry out inappropriate examinations. Equally, they must suggest modifications or alternatives to an examination when necessary. But, to do so, radiographers require both thorough knowledge and courage.

CONCLUSION

The importance of the practical radiation protection measures in relation to minimizing radiation dose during radiographic examinations has been discussed. In addition, the thoroughness of radiographers' knowledge about radiation protection has been questioned. Some of the matters raised might be considered by some to be peripheral to the everyday practice requirements of radiographers. However, this view does not accord with the requirements of the ionizing radiations legislation and radiographers have a clear role, and duty, to reduce the radiation dose at all times. However, the profession currently falls into two categories:

1. Those with their heads in the sand ignoring all but the basic requirements of their day-to-day work.
2. Those with foresight, who are looking to professional development and the fulfilment of a much broader role.

More radiographers must place themselves in the latter category, particularly in this critical area of radiation protection. Only by accepting this type of responsibility can radiographers move forward from a firm professional base to the next stages of development of their profession.

References

Calverd, A. (1993) Installation and subsequent testing. Poster presented at the Commission of the European Community Workshop in Dosimetry and Quality Assurance, Grado, Italy, September 1993.

College of Radiographers (1992) *Guidelines for the Introduction of a Quality Assurance Programme in a Diagnostic Imaging Department*. London: College of Radiographers.

Hawkes, N. (1991) 'Unnecessary X-rays blamed for up to 250 deaths per year.' *The Guardian*, 6 September.

Hughes, D. (1991) *Notes on Ionising Radiation: Biological Effects, Quantities, Dose Limits and Regulations*. HHSC Handbook No 8. Leeds: H & H Scientific Consultants.

Ionizing Radiations Regulations (1985). London: HMSO.

Ionizing Radiations (Protection of Persons Undergoing Medical Examinations or Treatment) Regulations (1988). London: HMSO.

NRPB (1988) *Guidelines for the Protection of Persons Against Ionizing Radiations Arising from Medical or Dental Use*. Didcot, UK: National Radiological Protection Board.

NRPB (1989) *Living with Radiation*, Vol. 1, no. 3. London: HMSO.

NRPB (1993) *Patient Dose Reduction in Diagnostic Radiology*, Vol. 1. Didcot, UK: National Radiological Protection Board.

NRPB and Royal College of Radiologists (1990) *Dose Limitation in Diagnostic Radiology*. Didcot, UK: National Radiological Protection Board.

Shrimpton, P. C., Wall, B. F., Jones, D. G. et al. (1986) *A National Survey of Doses to Patients Undergoing a Selection of Routine X-ray Examinations in English Hospitals (Chilton NRPB R200)*. London: HMSO.

X-rays. *Which?*, January 1991, p 40–41.

10

Audit of Professional Practice

Neil Prime

INTRODUCTION

The purpose of this chapter is to discuss the place that audit has in the practice of radiography. An overview is given of the development of audit, with its move from medical to clinical audit, together with its current and future applications. As will be shown, clinical audit is an essential part of the process of development of any profession. It helps in the growth of the profession, aids in business development and facilitates the educative processes. To not take part in audit or to not use audit as a tool in monitoring professional practice will retard the current development of radiography.

THE MOVE TO CLINICAL AUDIT

Audit as a process became formalized within the National Health Service (NHS) through the introduction of *Working Paper 6* (NHS, 1989). This defined medical audit as 'the systematic, critical analysis of the quality of medical care, including the procedures used for diagnosis and treatment, the use of resources, and the resulting outcome and quality of life for the patient'. While the paper identified the audit process as something that doctors were required to participate in and lead, it was clear that any definition that included the review of resources and use of diagnostic tests would inevitably be widened to multiprofessional audit. The word 'clinical' has been substituted for 'medical' in a definition given in a recent publication (NHSTD, 1994).

The White Paper, in outlining the structure of the audit process, also drew attention to audit activities that predated its inception. These included the work carried out by the Royal College of Radiologists, who established working parties in the mid-1970s to look at the national use of radiological services (Godwin, 1994). This work culminated in the production of guidelines by the Royal College of Radiologists (1990).

With the launch of the working paper, hospitals, trusts and primary care through the early 1990s set about interpreting the audit process and implemented it in a variety of ways. The system usually comprised an audit committee with a majority medical membership who co-ordinated audit throughout the organization. A review of the development of medical audit by Brunel University and the King's Fund (Kerrison et al., 1993), confirmed that in the hospitals studied this pattern was broadly followed, with meetings being held at varying times and with varying attendance. The presence of nursing and therapy staff was less common, but more frequent than representatives from general management. This pattern continues broadly today. The report by Kerrison et al. also gave a number of recommendations, including the need to focus audit projects on their ability to change practice and to measure the outcomes of the treatment process.

The formal move to clinical audit began 2 years after the launch of medical audit, as government soon realized that for audit to be a success all members of the health-care team needed to be involved. The 'launch' of clinical audit did not follow the same pattern as medical audit, but developed in two main ways. The first was funding, with £17.7 million being given to nursing and therapy audit in England during the period 1991–1994. Similar funding mechanisms were used in the rest of the UK (von Degenberg, 1993); see Table 10.1.

Table 10.1   Allocation to medical and clinical audit in England (von Degenberg, 1993)

Financial year	Medical audit in hospital and community services (£ million)	Nursing and therapy audit (£ million)
1989–1991	28.0	Nil
1991–1992	48.8	2.3
1992–1993	42.1	7.2
1993–1994	41.9	8.2
Total	160.8	17.7

These resources were used to develop projects at unit and/or regional level. The second initiative was the release of a variety of publications outlining what clinical audit was to achieve. Thus, clinical audit was seen as:

1. Multi- rather than uni-professional (NHSTD, 1994).
2. Part of an organization-wide approach to quality and part of purchaser/provider activity (NHS Management Executive, 1993).
3. Part of other related activities, such as continuous quality improvement (CQI).
4. Total quality management (TQM).
5. Professional standard setting and radiation protection (Department of Health, 1994).

The Evolution of Clinical Audit (Department of Health, 1994) gave the most developed overview of the continued development of clinical audit. Thus the need to make audit into a multiprofessional activity which becomes an integrated part of the business of a trust or general practice was seen as central.

Overall, the move has been to resource the transition from medical audit to multiprofessional audit, with the team approach being promoted to improve the delivery of health care.

WHAT IS THE AUDIT OF PROFESSIONAL PRACTICE?

Clinical audit is viewed as a cyclical process (Figure 10.1), and is described as such in many publications, for example *Making Medical Audit Effective* (Joint Centre for Education in Medicine, 1992). The process relies on the setting of standards at the beginning of the cycle. Practice is then measured against these standards and the outcome of the audit is a measure of the level of compliance with the standards. In some cases, the audit may reveal a gap between the standards and the processes for which they were set. Audit thus indicates areas for change to improve practice and the resulting change is re-audited as the cycle repeats itself.

In reality, the process is often not as simple as described. Difficulties may be encountered in the focusing of projects and the definition or development of standards and other outcome measures. Standards may not have been developed for areas of practice under consideration and audits are often undertaken as part-standard development/part-audit process.

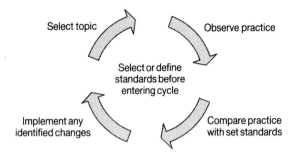

Figure 10.1   The audit cycle.

However, whatever the level of availability of standards, or the focus for the audit, clinical audit considers all aspects of the work of professionals and is therefore synonymous with the audit of professional practice. Audit is the tool for the review of how well professionals practise and how well they meet the needs of their clients. Clinical audit is focused on multiprofessional and collaborative audit and involves both professional and non-professional staff.

Clinical audit is not yet as well developed as medical audit. However, some professions are using systems such as the Dynamic Standard Setting System (DySSSy) (Royal College of Nursing, 1990), to develop standards which may be used to drive the audit cycle, while others are applying standard outcome measures to monitor the efficacy of available treatment (Mawson, 1993).

WHAT DO PROFESSIONALS AUDIT?

A review of common CD ROM databases such as *Health* (1975–July 1994) or *Cinahl* (1982–June 1994) reveals a broad range of audit activity. Subject areas include:

1. Record keeping and the accuracy of note/report writing.
2. Assessment of treatments through the use of outcome measures.
3. Assessment of specific treatment plans or clinical problems.
4. The use of audit in contracting and quality-assurance initiatives.
5. Discharge planning.
6. Client satisfaction with service provided.

The above areas account for the majority of subjects to which clinical audit has been applied. The spread of topics amongst professional groups broadly follows the numbers of professionals within each group, with nursing dominating the number of audits completed. A search of *Cinahl* and *Health* shows that 50% of recorded audits were nursing based, while specialities such as social work, physiotherapy and occupational therapy accounted for the remaining 50%. Radiography showed no recorded audit projects at all.

Other sources show a similar trend. A review of clinical audit carried out by the nursing and therapy professions in 1992–1993 (von Degenberg, 1994) revealed a predominance of nursing audit. Of the 356 clinical audit projects listed, radiography recorded only 2 (Table 10.2). Of the two projects recorded, the first shows only a minor role for the radiography department, while the second is listed as having had its funding withdrawn.

Table 10.2 Radiography audit projects 1992–1993 (von Degenberg, 1994)

Topic	Subject	Region of Origin
X-ray department audit	Multidisciplinary audit to provide seamless care for the discharge of the elderly to the community	Northern
Clients requiring radiotherapy	To audit the use of radiotherapy treatment	Yorkshire

This lack of radiographic audit activity may lead to the conclusion that radiographers do not carry out audit. This is not the case. However, a number of factors must be considered before concluding where radiographers stand in relation to clinical audit. The first is the relationship that radiographers have to medical audit. A report published on medical audit activity in hospital and community services (Stern and Brennan, 1994) lists audit activity by speciality. Diagnostic radiology has completed 157 medical audits while radiotherapy has completed 10 of the 2974 projects listed. The subjects audited in these specialities include:

1. The development or use of protocols and guidelines.
2. The appropriate use of specific examinations.
3. Outcomes of examinations.
4. Client satisfaction.
5. Departmental processes.

The range of topics listed is wide and many may be regarded as multiprofessional rather than medical audit. Examples such as

'Workload in main department'; 'Skin entrance doses for low kVp chest radiography'; 'Film rejects' and 'Computed tomography lumbar spine technique and interpretation in radiotherapy' illustrate this point. Each of these projects required significant input from radiographers. Hence, it appears that there is a well-developed clinical audit process with multiprofessional audit in place. But is it? The chances are it probably is not. Clinical audit has developed within radiology in a different way from its development in other professions such as physiotherapy. Radiography audit has evolved out of medical audit, whereas physiotherapy audit evolved as a free-standing method.

The second factor to be considered is the role of quality assurance in radiography. A return to the CD ROM soon generates a range of topics under the heading 'Quality and radiography', and the search reveals subject areas such as 'Inconsistencies in film processing quality' and 'Quality assurance in simulators'. There is thus widespread interest in quality issues and an awareness of quality. Why, then, has this not led to the development of clinical audit projects in radiography? Obviously, as was noted above, in some cases it has, and reject analysis is a good application of the audit cycle. However, the lack of spread of audit as a quality assurance tool in radiography must, again, be due to the way audit developed within the radiology/radiography field, with the initial growth of medical audit slowing the link between clinical audit and quality assurance.

THE FUTURE OF CLINICAL AUDIT IN RADIOGRAPHY

What is the future of clinical audit in radiography? As a quality method, the audit process will remain in place and will continue to develop. This is spelt out clearly in publications both from government and in the numerous quality journals available currently. Perhaps, more importantly, it is also the message coming from the health-care purchasers who perceive clinical audit to be 'the only process which can address effectively the evaluation of the clinical care of patients and show how standards and outcomes are being improved' (Coomber, 1994). This belief has already seen the inclusion of areas to be audited within contracts and service specifications agreed with providers. Over time, these inclusions will no doubt become more prescriptive, in line with the maturing of the health-care contracting process.

Clinical audit will also continue to act as a unifying force on the many strands and tools of quality assurance that are developing within the NHS. TQM, benchmarking (the comparison of standards between trusts), the critical-incident technique (CIT) and other initiatives all rely on and are being used in the audit process. Clinical audit is thus both a method and a culture which professionals and non-professionals alike need to develop.

The continued growth of audit will mean its application to an increasing number of areas of professional practice. These include:

1. *Patient-focused care*. With the writing of protocols and anticipated recovery pathways associated with patient-focused care, clinical audit is seen as an excellent tool for monitoring the success or failure of such schemes (Morgan, 1993). The involvement of radiographers here is in the debate over multiskilling and inclusion in treatment pathways. The impact of training professionals in a variety of roles on existing standards may be measured by clinical audit. Clinical audit will also help test the outcome of treatment and diagnosis.
2. *Contracting*. Here, explicitly, the clinical audit process will monitor performance against contracts.
3. *Patient satisfaction*. The continued development of the Patient's Charter and related league tables will demand the continued use of clinical audit.

The potential applications of audit to radiography are therefore vast, a fact confirmed at a recent series of workshops where radiographers of both specialities were asked to brainstorm ideas for audit (Prime, 1993). Delegates managed to develop 220 suggestions for audit without significant duplication. Table 10.3 gives an example of the combined

Table 10.3   Top 10 ideas generated by radiographers for clinical audit (Prime, 1993)

1	An audit of the use of lateral lumbar spines for patients referred by general practitioners
2	Monitoring patient waiting times following radiotherapy treatment
3	An audit of referrals for barium studies
4	An audit of the use of protocols in radiotherapy treatment
5	Waiting times prior to treatment/examination
6	Extending the role of radiographers
7	The use of guidelines in accident and emergency departments
8	Client satisfaction
9	A review of skull radiography in the department
10	Turn around times for reports

top 10 topics generated by two groups. As a whole, the suggested topics covered the following areas:

Contract monitoring   20%
Quality assurance   20%
Clinical areas   30%
Specialist topics   10%
Organizational audit   20%

The recognition that clinical audit may be applied to areas of radiography is thus well advanced.

CONCLUSION AND RECOMMENDATIONS

The use of clinical audit to monitor professional practice is recognized by radiographers but is poorly developed. This is due to the development of medical audit and quality assurance within radiology and radiotherapy which, particularly in its early stages, failed to recognize the contributions of radiographers.

The way forward must be the continued development of clinical audit by radiographers, to reflect both the interest in clinical audit shown by purchasers and the developing audit/quality culture within the NHS. This must not be uniprofessional but must encompass radiologists, nurses and other health workers as part of clinical, and not simply medical, audit. This process will happen through an increase in awareness of clinical audit and this may be facilitated by:

1. The establishment of a national database for radiographic clinical audit to share ideas, network, organize training and link with other databases.
2. The involvement of radiographers in audit training, both locally and nationally (see for example, University of Dundee (1994)).
3. The development of workshops and study days.
4. The development of links with other professionals conducting audit.

Finally, whatever direction the radiography profession moves in, and however radiography develops, there is no doubt that clinical audit is here to stay and must form a fundamental part of all radiographers' roles.

References

Cinahl (1982–June 1994). Glendale: Cinahl Information Services.

Coomber, G. (1994) The purchaser's view. In Hopkins, A. (ed.) *Professional and Managerial Aspects of Clinical Audit*. London: Royal College of Physicians.

Department of Health (1994) *The Evolution of Clinical Audit*. Leeds: NHS Management Executive.

Godwin, R. (1994) Royal College of Radiologists. In Hopkins, A. (ed.) *Professional and Managerial Aspects of Clinical Audit*, pp 47–51. London: Royal College of Physicians.

Health (1975–July 1994). Bethesda, MD: National Library of Medicine.

Joint Centre for Education in Medicine (1992) *Making Medical Audit Effective*. London: Joint Centre for Education in Medicine.

Kerrison, S., Packwood, T., Buxton, M. (1993) *Medical Audit – Taking Stock*. London: Brunel University/King's Fund Centre.

Mawson, S.T. (1993) Measuring physiotherapy outcome in stroke rehabilitation. *Physiotherapy* **79:** 762–765.

Morgan, G. (1993) The implications of patient focused care. *Nursing Standard* **7:** 37–39.

NHS (1989) *Working for Patients – Medical Audit (Working Paper 6)*. London: HMSO.

NHS Management Executive (1993) *EL(93)116 – Achieving an Organisation Wide Approach to Quality*. Leeds: NHS Management Executive.

NHSTD (1994) *Getting Ahead with Clinical Audit – A Facilitator's Guide*. London: NHS Management Executive, NHSTD.

Prime, N. (1993) A Clinical Audit Workshop Workbook. Unpublished.

Royal College of Nursing (1990) *Quality Patient Care – The Dynamic Standard Setting System*. London: Royal College of Nursing.

Royal College of Radiologists (1990) *Making the Best Use of a Department of Radiology. Guidelines for Doctors*. London: Royal College of Radiologists.

Stern, M., Brennan, S. (1994) *Medical Audit in the Hospital and Community Health Service*. London: Department of Health.

University of Dundee (1994) *Moving to Audit*. Dundee: Centre for Medical Education, Ninewells Hospital and Medical School.

von Degenberg, K. (1994) *Clinical Audit in The Nursing and Therapy Professions*. London: Department of Health.

11

Digital Imaging – State of the Art and Future Potential

Andrew Todd-Pokropek

INTRODUCTION

Film, as used in radiology, is a remarkable medium. It has a large dynamic range; it has a very high information capacity; it is (relatively) cheap; it can be used wherever there is a source of light; it is very flexible (both physically and in range of use). Digital displays have a poor dynamic range, a low information capacity, are expensive, cannot easily be moved, and impose new patterns of use in a health-care environment. Why therefore are so many of us trying to replace film by digital computer-driven displays? Are there real clinical advantages which become feasible using digital imaging methods, or is it just fashion, as some people claim about the use of (audio) compact discs with respect to vinyl records?

Part of the answer lies in the ability, using digital systems, to separate the image from its support, distinguishing the image data from the picture that is viewed. The current state of the art of the use of digital images is certainly limited; however, the future potential is very important not only in that it should facilitate new methods of extracting clinical information, but also considerable changes in working practice are likely. In this chapter one view of this is described, postulating how it is possible to go from the present position in radiology to where it should be in the not too distant future.

WHAT IS DIGITAL IMAGING?

In the loose sense, digital imaging is any imaging procedure which has as its result the production of an image in digital form. In that sense, computed tomography (CT) and magnetic resonance imaging (MRI), the use of photostimulable plates in computerized radiology (CR), digital subtraction angiography (DSA) and much nuclear medicine (NM) can be considered forms of digital imaging, while conventional film-based radiography is not. However, this is cheating in a way. Most radiologists seem to report CT images from film, and not from the computer screen (the so-called 'soft copy'), and most current CT systems seem to be treated as digital devices, for creating analogue film. This is not really digital imaging in the sense intended. It is rather like the comparison of analogue cellular telephones with the new (GSM) digital telephones where there is little external difference apparent in the quality of the reproduction of the voice, although there is considerable difference in the way in which the voice information is transmitted.

So why is digital imaging so exciting? Some of the reasons are functional, relating to the way in which the images can be used in practice; some reasons are fundamental, concerning the kind of information which could be used. The first obvious feature of a digital image is that it can be modified; for example, the windowing can be changed, the image can be zoomed, and the grey scale or colour scale can be changed. The good result of this is that low-contrast features are easier to detect in digital images. The bad result is that it takes longer to interpret a digital image on soft copy (a screen) than on film, and/or more images are generally produced.

A second obvious feature of a digital image is that it can be copied, it can be sent to several places at the same time and, in principle, it cannot be lost. While the loss of films is well known and usually a result of bad practice (the borrower of the film forgetting to return it), the loss of digital data is also well known as a result of bad practice (pouring coffee over a floppy disk, dropping a large optical disk, etc.). In both cases, good practice must be encouraged to prevent loss, in which case, the digital system has significant advantages.

A potential advantage of a digital imaging system is that the reporting of images can be facilitated and, in principle, the result of a test can be available faster than with conventional film. This is not an automatic benefit, but one that can be achieved by changes in working practice. A corresponding advantage is that, potentially, the matching of images to patients can be improved, in particular with respect to old images.

Finally, the kind of information available from digital images can be improved. Interpretation is currently often very subjective, the use of image processing can add objective information. Using digital images, measurements can be made. These measurements could be valueless (the angle of the patient's nose) or valuable, for example the change in volume of a tumour over a course of treatment. In addition, images from different sources can be superimposed (registration) and displayed together (fusion), making available a range of new techniques; these are so far unused (and untested).

WHAT IS THE CURRENT STATE OF THE ART?

This subject may be divided into the following areas:

1. Acquisition.
2. Image transmission.
3. Display.
4. Archiving.
5. Handling associated data.

Acquisition

To replace conventional film, the best candidate at present is the CR plate. The CR plates in use have a resolution of 2000 × 2000 (about 3–5 line pairs per millimetre), excellent linearity, 'equivalent' sensitivity to film (a subject worth a paper in its own right) and are relatively slow to read out, typically taking 1–2 minutes. Progress is possible; using thinner plates, or by similar modification, the resolution can be doubled, but read-out is slower. Speed could be improved by using multiple lasers, but cost would increase. The use of other materials or detectors is not excluded, for example large charge coupled device (CCD) arrays. It seems likely that, within the next few years, a number of detectors with resolution comparable to film will be available, with an improved effective performance in terms of sensitivity, linearity and dynamic range. Film digitization currently lags behind, where state-of-the-art digitizers have a performance comparable to, but slightly worse than, current CR systems.

Acquisition by pure digital systems, in particular MRI, is likely to increase and, as it has in the past, encroach on a number of new areas, such as interventional radiology and in vitro imaging (MRI and ultrasound microscopy). New methods are likely to be developed, for example applied potential tomography, optical spectroscopy and tomography. Such systems will interface easily with current digital systems. In summary, digital acquisition should be available for all practical applications.

Image Transmission

Here the state of the art used to be the ethernet cable, with a capacity of 10 Mbit s^{-1} capable, in theory, of transferring a digital X-ray in about 10 s. Improvements by factors of 10 have been achieved. Using fibre-optic cables within a hospital (FDDI), transfer speeds of 100 Mbit s^{-1} and greater are available. The new Asynchronous Transmission Mode (ATM) standard permits transfer rates of 34 Mbit s^{-1} anywhere (one hospital to another, one country to another) and higher speed networks are being worked on. The 'infobahn' is a reality, and problems in image transmission will become a thing of the past. All that is needed is to find the money to install the necessary cabling and interfaces.

Actually, this is not quite true, and there is still a bottleneck in getting the images onto and off the network. Computers currently cannot work as fast as the networks that are available. However this, too, is in the process of being rectified using large parallel magnetic disk systems (RAIDs), although the associated costs are not negligible.

There are currently good standards for methods of transmitting images between different systems, in particular, DICOM (NEMA, 199X), and INTERFILE in nuclear medicine (Todd-Pokropek et al., 1992).

Display

The display of digital images is still, relatively, the weak point of a digital imaging system. Displays capable of displaying 1000 × 1000 pixels are commonplace, and not quite adequate for high resolution, difficult radiological images. Displays of 2000 × 2000 pixels are expensive, not very bright, and not very satisfactory. An unanswered question is whether displays with lower resolution than the images themselves (using a 1000 × 1000 pixel display with a 2000 × 2000 pixel CR image) provide adequate clinical performance, or whether it degrades the system. While this is currently a 'religious' question, it is likely to be answered by a number of the large scale picture archiving and communication system (PACS) prototypes.

An associated question is: How many displays are needed at one time? This is limited by the cost of the display and, probably more importantly, by the amount of space available. Current display systems are relatively slow, rather cumbersome and, overall, not very satisfactory. In addition, since there is a tendency to place many displays in the hospital or health-care network, the cost as well as the poor performance is multiplied by a potentially large factor.

It is suggested that, with the advent of the new high-quality television standards, this problem might disappear, as large numbers of cheap televisions of suitable quality might become available. Other systems such as liquid crystal devices (LCDs), projectors, screens, and even eye glasses might provide alternative solutions.

Archiving

As with networks, the progress with respect to storing digital images has been spectacular. If it is assumed that a digital X-ray requires 4 Mbyte of storage, devices capable of storing up to 1 million such images are almost commonplace, and remarkably inexpensive. Costs of about 20 pence (US$ 0.3) per image are current on optical disks, but factors of 10 or more can easily be achieved to reduce this.

An alternative storage method that should be considered is the use of smart cards (similar to credit cards with storage) to be retained by the patients. It will soon be feasible, but not necessarily desirable, for all radiological images to be given back to the patient for them to look after, or lose, themselves, rather than the hospital. An alternative scenario is that all images through the world are stored in a centralized archive (under the Pentagon in Washington?). Neither scenario – total dispersion or total centralization – is likely to come true. Most probably there will be a similar situation to that currently experienced; multiple copies of data, missing data, misplaced data, mislabelled data or, in other words, a fuzzy system. The major task with an archiving system is to be able to locate and handle such a fuzzy system in an efficient and clinically satisfactory manner.

Handling Associated Data

The most important type of associated data is the patient demographic information: who the patient is, how they can be contacted, and how billing can be performed. This information is not in the province of radiology. The most difficult current task in the implementation of large-scale PACSs has been in the interfacing of the radiology system with the other hospital computers (MIMOSA Consortium, 1994). This is likely to become even more important as the provision of health care devolves increasingly into the community. In this case there is a good solution: the adoption of appropriate standards, such that the exchange of information between many different types of systems can be facilitated, and that the data exchanged can be understood. This has important implications not only at the European level, in terms of translation between different languages, but also in the important task of creating clinical records which can be understood by different clinicians, that is, the use of appropriate terminology.

PILOT INSTALLATIONS

There are two types of installation of digital imaging networks which have been tried: small-scale mini-PACS (sneakernets) and large-scale hospital-wide systems to enable filmless hospitals to be tested. Good examples of the latter (*c.* 1994) are at the Hammersmith Hospital London (Allison et al., 1994), the Danube Hospital Vienna (Hruby, 1994), and the MDIS system in the USA. There are a great many examples of the former type of installation.

The initial pilot studies were, clinically, very disappointing, and the systems were slow and difficult to use, and provided unsatisfactory image quality. They showed that while the basic ideas might be correct, the technical state of the art lagged behind, a situation which took much longer to advance than was originally suspected. There is a joke where a computer scientist was asked how long a task would take. He replied that it would take only a couple of computer minutes (where each computer minute is composed of an unknown number of computer seconds).

However, while the success of these large-scale installations remains to be proven, it is clear that there has been enormous progress in that it is now, just about, technically feasible to run a filmless hospital, even if it may not be cheap. The recent claims from, for example, the Danube hospital about the reduction of reporting time, and hence patient stay, seem to be convincing.

The success of the small-scale installations is also clear. It is becoming increasingly difficult to visit a radiology department which has both a CT and an MRI system without at least having the question asked: How can they be connected together? Every manufacturer of such systems now claims that they have, or will soon have, connection using DICOM or, in nuclear medicine, INTERFILE. The associated costs, in terms of equipment, can be remarkably small. A network of four Unix workstations can be installed for less than £20 000 (US$30 000). However, such systems require an expert physicist or programmer to support them, at a non-negligible cost. The major task of such systems is now to cross the frontier from research to clinical routine.

CHANGES IN WORKING PRACTICE

Digital images are likely to be much more readily available outside the radiology department than are films. Working practice will change with the availability of radiological images; for example, in intensive care, transmitting the images back to the bedside using the same systems as are currently used for monitoring. The question of responsibility for reporting is an issue. Should images be released from radiology before reporting? Should clinicians outside the service department be permitted to report? What is the function of an imaging service such as radiology? The practices in different countries are dissimilar. In Japan, for example, much reporting is performed by the referring physician. This is the so-called 'turf' dispute. There is a strong and increasing incentive for referring clinicians to do their own interpretation and reporting, when that is permitted. Since the referring clinicians have the patients, in the long term they have the necessary clout to make this happen, unless there is a good reason to continue present practice. It is clear that, in some areas at least, perhaps cardiology for example, service departments such as radiology will lose out, unless they can provide additional clinical value that the referring services cannot obtain or provide otherwise. This implies a change in working practice.

Designing and implementing a PACS network implies that the mechanisms for reporting be modelled, and an electronic reporting system be created, as has been reported by the MIMOSA group. There is no reason to mimic current practice. Thus the role of an imaging department in terms of how its routine workload is managed could change dramatically, presumably with the aim of improving efficiency and, possibly, reducing staff.

In addition, the availability of digital image data from different modalities means that it is relatively easy to combine them, that is to put together different types of images, for example CT and MRI, or nuclear medicine and angiography. The registration of such data to ensure that they are accurately positioned, and the formation of composite or hybrid images (so-called 'image fusion') and their processing to extract quantitative information is an important area of research (Todd-Pokropek, 1994). There is considerable potential for the extraction of additional clinical information by using such techniques. Thus there is an argument to suggest that the role of an imaging service such as radiology may become more concerned with the extraction of clinical information from a variety of combined imaging modalities, rather than being merely the technical provider of basic images. The role would change from being a clinical 'photographer' to becoming a graphic studio/audiovisual centre, by analogy. Thus, image processing, manipulation and management could make available new ways of improving clinical performance.

Finally, the ability to transmit images over long distances means that the way in which clinical services are currently provided could change. There could be a shift with respect to where particular types of imaging procedures take place – in a hospital service or in the community. An example might be in the provisions to be made for keyhole surgery. Also, the way in which clinical experts are made available throughout the health system could change, for example in the provision of neuroradiologists for MRI, or of paediatric radiologists with respect to district general hospitals.

In the same way as there has been considerable change in the way that health care is funded, it is very likely that the way in which imaging services are provided and reported will change, both in terms of the types of examination which are performed, and in the way in which clinical information is provided. The availability of facilities for handling digital image data will serve as a mechanism for facilitating such change. However, one thing that is almost certain is that the type of staff employed within a service such as radiology will change as the expertise required of them alters.

CONCLUSION – THE FUTURE

As has been said above, it is very difficult to make predictions, especially about the future. It seems likely that digital imaging will become current and dominate routine radiology in the middle future –

the next 10 years. The implication that accompanies this is that radiological practice will change significantly. The tendency to subspecialization in radiology is likely to increase; clinically, radiologists can only add value if they are clinically highly competent in the appropriate domain (Rinck, 1994). If, for example, a referring cardiologist cannot understand the cardiological information that a radiologist is trying to convey, if that radiologist is not convincing, then confidence will not be established, and eventually, the radiologist imager will be bypassed.

The idea of a radiologist being an expert medical 'photographer' is likely to pass into history; the idea of a specialist radiologist expert in the particular clinical speciality and familiar with all the relevant imaging modalities is likely to become the norm. Who then provides the imaging and instrumental expertise? Not the radiologist, but presumably the radiographer, and the radiological instrumental specialist. There is a need both to educate this new type of specialist (who might be a radiographer, or a physicist, or a computer scientist or a mixture of all three) and for radiologists to 'retrain' and to form better links with clinical specialities. The pattern both of performing the imaging procedure and reporting seems bound to change.

These changes will take some time to happen, but preparing for them should start now. This means changes in roles and function of members of the radiology department, facilitated by further education. The use of multimodality image fusion, and extraction of quantitative data from radiological images, while currently of unproven clinical value, remains as a major tool for improving clinical benefit from digital imaging procedures.

References

Allison, D.J., Marin, N.J., Reynolds, R.A. et al. (1994) Clinical aspect of PACS. In Tan, L., Siew, E. (eds) *Proceedings of the 18th International Congress of Radiology (ICR94)*, Singapore, January 1994, pp 813–819.

Hruby, W. (1994) Digital radiology: integration of HIS-RIS-PACS. Two years clinical experience. Presented in *Post-Congress Meeting, Picture Archiving and Documentation Systems in Nuclear Medicine – An Impact on Quality of Patient Care.* Münster, Germany, August 1994.

MIMOSA Consortium (1994) Medical image management in an open system architecture, the mimosa models. European Project AIM A2009, workpackage WP3 M/WP3/VUB/1, March 1994.

NEMA (199X) Digital imaging and communications in medicine, Parts 1–10. *NEMA Standards Publication PS3.2.* NEMA.

Rinck, P.A. (1994) Do radiologists have a future? *Diagnostic Imaging International*, Sept.: 19–20.

Todd-Pokropek, A. (1994) PACS: from research to clinical reality. BIR Annual Lecture, Harrogate, May 1994.

Todd-Pokropek, A., Cradduck, T.D., Deconinck, F. (1992) A file format for the exchange of nuclear medicine image data: a specification of Interfile version 3.3. *Nuclear Medicine Communications* **13:** 673–699.

12

Computed Radiography – the Conquest Experience

David Baker

INTRODUCTION

At the time of writing, the Conquest Hospital in Hastings, Sussex, has been open for 15 months. During the design stages of the hospital, an undertaking was made to develop a picture archive and communication system (PACS) for the radiology department. The funding for this project would come from South East Thames Regional Health Authority (Foord, 1993).

The name of the system under design became known as the 'intelligent local area network' (iLAN). A major portion of the iLAN project at the Conquest Hospital is the computed radiography (CR) segment. To date, this segment has been used for soft-copy viewing (i.e. viewing plain radiographs on a computer screen) within the accident and emergency (A&E) department and for soft-copy reporting (i.e. reporting plain radiographs from a computer screen) within radiology for more than a year.

For the purposes of this work, the CR segment may be defined as that equipment which generates, and displays digital plain radiographs, be that in the wet processing area, in the A&E department or the radiologist's reporting room. Its use on an operational basis began in mid-1993 and since then certain challenges have arisen. Such challenges may be grouped under training, ergonomics, and quality.

TRAINING

So far, staff groups that have undergone training have included radiographers, radiologists, A&E nurses and medical staff and support staff such as clerical officers and dark-room technicians. Each group had its own unique training requirements and most training was on a one-to-one or one-to-two basis.

Training requirements were established by taking each staff group in turn, by examining what old activities would disappear when CR replaced portions of conventional radiography and what new activities would be needed to replace them. Their functional relation with other tasks carried out by each staff group, and those tasks which together would form the whole process of imaging handling, were then examined (Dalla Palma et al., 1992).

For example, as regards radiographers, they would not be using the conventional methods of developing images, which at the Conquest was a daylight processor used to develop latent images acquired on a film, with the aid of a cassette and intensifying screens. Instead, they would use the Fuji photostimulable phosphor plates and the Philips ACe Plate Reader. In essence, this involved having a cassette loaded with a phosphor plate, examining the patient in the usual manner and then feeding the plate into the plate reader. The latent image would be acquired by the plate-reader software and then displayed on a computer screen prior to archiving and sending to other departments. These training needs for radiographers were recognized readily.

The allocation of new tasks to A&E and support staff and therefore the establishment of training needs was more subtle. It is still an ongoing process. For example, A&E nurses were recognized as a significant asset when it came to managing the A&E workstation, given the fact that the turnover of nursing staff is much lower than that of casualty officers. Teaching this staff group image display skills would reduce the urgency for training every casualty officer on the first day of their new job. Previously, nurses would not have been so involved in managing radiographs within their department, and hence a whole new role developed for nurses.

Initial application training was given by the suppliers of the iLAN software and hardware, SIMIS Medical Imaging and Philips, the supplier of the ACe Plate Reader. A small core of senior radiographers and superintendent radiographers was targeted in this initial training. The knowledge derived from the training of this small core was worked into a holistic form and cascaded in a single tier to members of the staff groups mentioned previously.

Such training was labour intensive. However, in the medium term it minimized the need to deal with low-level fault finding.

Competence Requirements

Radiologists were required to be competent in the following tasks:

1. Calling up images either preloaded onto their workstation for reporting or making ad hoc enquiries.
2. Manipulating images, including such features as optical density, contrast and edge enhancement.
3. Undertaking minor troubleshooting.

It took 2–4 reporting sessions to reach competence in these tasks.

Radiographers' skills were required to match the following:

1. Use of the Philips ACe system and Fuji CR plates to obtain the best possible images with the lowest patient dose.
2. Manipulation of the image at the CR workstation and transmission to iLAN and, if necessary, to another soft-copy address.
3. Printing of hard-copy images from the 3M laser imager for those areas not equipped with a view station.
4. Undertaking minor and intermediate troubleshooting for their own and all other staff groups.

This training requirement was addressed with tutorials and 2–4 sessions of supervised plain radiography, starting with simple chest examinations and working up to more complex and improvised trauma work. It is important to emphasize, however, that the learning, and the passing on of lessons in relation to such a new way of working is never-ending.

A&E staff were required to:

1. Receive images direct from the CR view station to their own view station.
2. Display the appropriate images.
3. If necessary, manipulate the images for optimum viewing.

New doctors within this department coped well with this unique experience, not having had sufficient exposure to conventional methods to have experienced culture shock. Less recently qualified doctors took longer to acclimatize.

Nurses coped well with image retrieval. This staff group had only recently undergone training on a new hospital information system (HIS) and were getting used to work practices associated with new technology. Within 4–6 weeks, nursing staff became self-sufficient in looking after their part of the segment.

Training does need periodic reinforcement and this, in itself, places a burden on staff using the system, especially once the vendor companies have gone.

Support staff were required to be competent in the following range of tasks:

1. Establishing whether an image is present on the network.
2. Building folders for pre-sending onto the radiologist workstation in good time for reporting.
3. Alerting either a radiographer or darkroom technician to those images that require hard copying, i.e. printing from the 3M laser imager.

This group became competent in these functions in approximately 5 working days.

Automated folder building of preloaded images is planned for the long term, whilst in the short term a dedicated reporting room is being constructed with a higher specification workstation to make better use of reporting sessions.

Early in 1994, the system was shut down for a period of 3 weeks, for reconfiguring to a more efficient format. One of the effects of this shutdown was the loss of some of the skills acquired by all staff groups during the operational period up to that point. Refresher training was required and, at this point in time, this demand, together with a not unreasonable scepticism on the part of staff, must be seen as a consequence of a multistaged development project being employed in an operational role.

ERGONOMICS

There is need for evidence of an improvement in the efficiency of operation before PACSs are to find widespread use. Therefore, once training was complete, the effect of the new working patterns required assessment.

Radiologists reported during their timetabled sessions. Certain radiologists had lower specification workstations than others and efficiency was impaired in these situations by as much as a factor of 3. This is being addressed with a dedicated digital reporting room, the success of which is yet to be determined. The older models will be sent out to those areas earmarked for expansion where retrieval time is not such a crucial factor, for example chest clinics.

Reporting was found to be cumbersome when performed in conjunction with paper request forms. There are plans to incorporate digitized request forms within the patient's folio of images.

Radiographers began using CR with general practitioner referrals and expanded in a short period to A&E work.

Prior to this changeover, a study was undertaken into the well-recognized bottleneck that occurred at the daylight processor, when during busy periods latent images are acquired faster than they can be processed. It was found that in 45% of processing episodes, there was another image awaiting development within 30 seconds following the commencement of the first processing episode. In 33% of cases, this initial episode was followed by another within 30–60 seconds and yet one more within 60–120 seconds. This study was carried out on a 3M Trim daylight loader and X515 processor, its output established at a level of 80 plates per hour. The output for the Philips ACe CR system was cited as 40 plates per hour in the manufacturer's literature; however, a practical level is lower than this.

It was anticipated that during busy periods work patterns would have to change from radiographers working singly or in pairs (staffing permitting) to one radiographer reviewing images and controlling the processing of plates whilst colleagues generated images only. This practice has not yet been perfected, as there needs to be a fine balance between using new technology and imposing new practices merely to address basic flaws in the efficiency of capital equipment.

In addition, an interface between the Philips ACe system and the departmental radiology information system is being designed. In the 1995–1996 financial year, another plate reader will also be purchased.

With regard to patient care as a whole, radiologists do not have to wait for images to return from A&E for reporting. Reporting is therefore more timely, presenting the opportunity for radiologists' reports to be used more effectively in the patient management process (Straub and Gur, 1990). This is particularly important in A&E when initial patient-management decisions may be based on a senior house officer's opinion of a radiograph.

IMAGE QUALITY

Once the image is scanned by the CR plate reader, the raw data are subject to processing by the Philips and Fuji software. There are three modes of operation. Fixed mode offers fixed latitude and sensitivity and is therefore akin to a conventional film–screen combination. Semi-mode has a fixed latitude but variable sensitivity. Auto-mode has both latitude and sensitivity flexibility, and is the mode routinely used. Of the images obtained, 90% are satisfactory.

To back up anecdotal evidence, an experiment was conducted to compare identical CR and conventional images. This was achieved by sandwiching a CR plate, an insulating sheet, and an intensifying screen within a conventional cassette. (The intensifying screen was of sufficient speed to match the performance of the two-screen format routinely used within the department.) Thus, by using routine exposures, CR and conventional images were obtained at no extra dose to the patient. Both images were viewed side by side, one on a viewing box and one on a workstation. By no means was this an attempt at an ROC survey. It did, however, confirm the findings of previous works (Fink et al., 1993; Frey et al., 1993). These have established that, although digital images have a lower spatial resolution than conventional ones, this is compensated for by the facility of image manipulation.

Of the images obtained, 10% required manipulation for optimum viewing, but among this group were certain examinations that the dynamic range of the system appeared to be unable to address. Such examinations were dorsiplantar feet, lateral lumbar spines and those projections in which the patient presented with a wide contrast range. Metal anatomical markers, by introducing further density ranges and edges, tended to exacerbate this feature in these examinations. To tackle this challenge, the tightest possible collimation, along with use of lead rubber at the margins of the radiation field, was employed, although this was impossible for certain trauma examinations. At present, SIMIS Medical Imaging are working on a gradient manipulation tool which will enable remapping of the image along a sensitometric curve more suited to the individual patient's contrast range. Philips have also recognized this as a problem and are introducing new software and hardware interfaces to their CR units. To reduce the impact that the anatomical markers may have on these images, a step wedge style marker is under design. Experimental work is being undertaken to determine the required material, thickness and steps.

Another problem with markers was discovered in periodic reject analysis surveys. In 1–4% of images markers were missing from the image, either through error or through the imaging processing problems mentioned above. Because the images cannot be marked subsequently, these examinations required repeating. Such repeats were offset by the virtual elimination of rejects due to errors in exposure. Work has therefore to be done into digital image annotation. Such a tool will also enable such remarks as 'expiration' and 'erect' to be recorded on the image.

CONCLUSION

A whole range of challenges have been encountered and are being dealt with. Although the use of such a raw product has at times caused operational difficulties, it has enabled the emergence of key issues which may not be encountered in the factory design stage.

To make the most of this new digital modality the main issues may be summarized as follows:

1. Recognition that there is a heavy ongoing training need within and without the department.
2. Provision needs to be made for unforeseen events and for development requirements. Indeed, the main unforeseen event at the Conquest was the disappearance of the Regional Health Authority along with its development funding. Hastings and Rother NHS Trust are, to the best of their abilities, funding further stages of the project in the expectation, on completion, there will be a viable, economic and qualitatively justified system.
3. To make the best of the large initial capital outlay that is entailed in purchasing any PACS hardware and software, changes in work practices for all groups of staff require close examination (Dalla Palma et al., 1992). This is not only important for maximum examination throughout, but also to ensure that staff do not serve the new technology. Rather, the technology must serve the staff and the patient.

References

Dalla Palma, L., Giribona, P., Stakul, F. et al. (1992) The Trieste PACS project. *Integrated Diagnostic Imaging*, pp 227–238, London: Elsevier.

Fink, V., Widmann, A., Fink, B.J. et al. (1993) Primary and secondary digitizing of X-ray images in comparison to conventional films. *Computer Assisted Radiology* **93:** 441–446.

Foord, K.D. (1993) The iLAN project in Hastings, UK: status in October 1993. *Europacs Newsletter* **Dec.:** 1.

Frey, G.D., Starr, C.W., Usher, L.B. (1993) Digital image quality: a contrast details study using the Leeds Phantom. *Computer Assisted Radiology* **93:** 83–88.

Straub, W.H., Gur, D. (1990) Hidden costs of delayed access to diagnostic imaging information: impact on PACS implementation. *American Journal of Roentgenology* **156:** 613–616.

13

Image Transmission and Picture Archiving and Communication Systems – the Potential

Nuala Martin and Anne Hemingway

INTRODUCTION

The nightmare scenario of a master computer which holds information about every aspect of our personal lives is not new and is a theme that has formed the basis of many works of science fiction. As sophisticated computer systems are introduced into the hospital environment, will patients and staff suffer the same plight as Orwell's characters or can the enormous potential of such systems be harnessed to improve the quality of service offered to patients? One thing is certainly true: like the rest of society, medicine is drowning in information; Stewart (1994) claims that more new information has been produced in the last 30 years than in the previous 5000, and the sum of all printed knowledge doubles every 8 years.

Those who work within the medical imaging field are in a more difficult situation than most in the rest of medicine and society because of the vast quantities of information contained within radiographic images. It used to be said that one picture is worth a thousand words, but in computer terms a complex radiographic image is worth not 1000 but 9 million words; one chest image holding the equivalent amount of digital information to the Old and the New Testaments of the Bible combined. The task, therefore, of developing computers and networks

niving and transmitting these data sets with a view to
m and paper records from radiology departments and
been little short of prodigious. There are, nevertheless, a
ure archiving and communication systems (PACSs) now
available which are capable of undertaking this task.
ld be capable not only of displaying current radiographic
so of storing, transmitting and displaying patient infor-
maging and demographic) from various modalities over
se of a patient's history of investigation. To achieve these
inges must take place in operational procedures and
structures to ensure the proper use of a PACS so that its
an be realized in terms of both diagnostic interpretation
ital management.
e divided into two broad categories based on their archi-

lized system.
ar system.

LIZED SYSTEM

designed to be hospital wide, with the intention of vir-
ting the use of all x-ray film (hard copy). Such a system
eing installed at Hammersmith Hospital and has been
llison et al. (1994). This particular system, shown in
onsists of a centralized store, called a working storage
vhich has 40 Gbyte of on-line magnetic storage. Images
ing 2:1 reversible compression and may be accessed
stations with retrieval times of the order of 2 seconds via
bre-optic link which is called an 'Imagenet'. The link is
star topology and is capable of transmitting image data
r second. The second network, the control network, is an
h transmits the demographic data to the workstation
irried with the image information at the time of display.
rage is provided by two Kodak Optical Disk Jukeboxes
14-inch optical disks; each jukebox is capable of storing
formation which will accommodate approximately 13
ie imaging data (Figure 13.2). Computed radiographic
will be compressed 10:1 irreversibly on the ODJs. All
vill be reversibly compressed at 2:1.

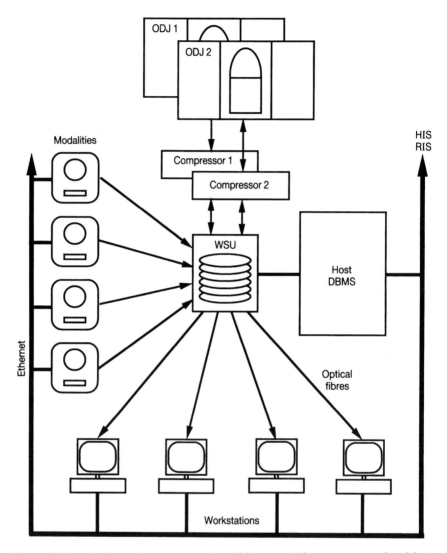

Figure 13.1   A schematic representation of the essential components of and their connections within a centralized PACS system (Hammersmith Hospital). DBMS, database management system; HIS, hospital information system; RIS, radiology information system; ODJ, optical disk jukebox; WSU, working storage unit.

The image display workstations are all monochrome screens and are based on Macintosh computers. There will be 151 workstations distributed throughout the hospital and of the 30 of these allocated to radiology, 6 will be for primary interpretation (Figure 13.3). There are two types of workstation:

1. *Diagnostic reporting workstations* (DRWs) which have a resolution of 1536 × 2048 pixels per screen and brightness of 275 cd m^{-2} with single, double or quadruple monitors attached. These will be used for primary diagnosis.
2. *Clinical review workstations* (CRWs) which have a resolution of 1052 × 882 pixels per screen and brightness of 200 cd m^{-2} with single or double monitors attached. These will be used for image review.

This system has been designed and developed under contract with Siemens Gammasonics Incorporated and Loral Western Development Laboratories. The development has taken place in close collaboration with the users to ensure a clinically useful system which enables an operator not only to view images but also to link them systematically with patients' demographic and report data. In order to maximize the clinical and research potential of stored images, the Hammersmith group have developed, with the manufacturers, a folder concept known as the Hammersmith Index of Folder Linked Images (HIFLI). This enables the radiographers, radiologists, clinicians and other groups of hospital personnel to organize patient data into subfolders, for example, modality, body part and conference (Figure 13.4). This acts as a filtering system to reduce information overload and provides rapid access to the information related to a particular patient, group of patients or modality.

THE MODULAR SYSTEM

A modular PACS is designed around the different functional imaging units found within a radiology department. The largest installation of this type is located at the Danube Hospital SMZ, Vienna, Austria (Greenacher and Berthold, 1994). The system shown in Figure 13.5 allows different clusters of imaging modalities to be connected to the fibre data distribution interface (FDDI) network. Each cluster has its own local storage unit (image storage and archiving (ISA)) which allows 3–5 modalities to be connected. For speed of access, current inpatient images are kept on a fast magnetic storage medium with a capacity of up to 35 Gbyte per ISA. After they have been reported, the images are stored using a reversible data compression factor of 2.5 : 1 on 5¼-inch optical disks. Jukeboxes for the disks enable 7 Gbyte of information to be stored on each ISA. The images are displayed on workstations which are based on SPARC2 architecture with 64 Mbyte to 1.7 Gbyte central processing unit (CPU) memory. Images which are stored within the cluster are available within 5 seconds at the workstations. The images are organized into imaging folders, but the capability does not exist at present for storing examination reports on the PACS or displaying them on the workstations.

The relative advantages and disadvantages of these two different PACSs are hotly contested and it will take many years of practical experience and debate to determine which, if either, is better; what is beyond question, however, is the fact that the purchase of either system will commit the institution concerned to revolutionary changes in the use of information technology.

INTERFACES

The main objective in the development of PACS interfaces has, to date, been to ensure that the equipment and modalities from different manufacturers can be interfaced into the system being developed. The difficulties surrounding this issue have been significantly underesti-

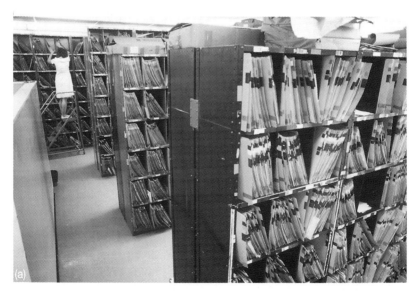

Figure 13.2   (a) A conventional film stack, storing just 15-months worth of x-ray film.

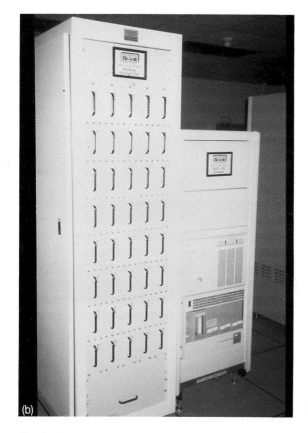

Figure 13.2   (b) A jukebox with the capacity to store up to 6-years worth of patient imaging data.

mated, particularly those relating to the integration of demographic data. The standards laid down by the American College of Radiologists and the National Electrical Manufacturing Association (ACR/NEMA) (version 2) did not adequately describe the required demographic leader data needed to ensure correct profiling within any PACS. The working party set up by this ACR/NEMA group has therefore developed a further interface standard known as the Digital Imaging and Communications in Medicine Standard (DICOM) (version 3) which addresses many of the problems related to the transmission of demographic data across networks (Bidgood and Horil, 1992). This standard was introduced at the Radiological Society of North America (RSNA) meeting in Chicago in 1993, but has yet to be accepted by all equipment manufacturers. There are many computers, particularly hospital

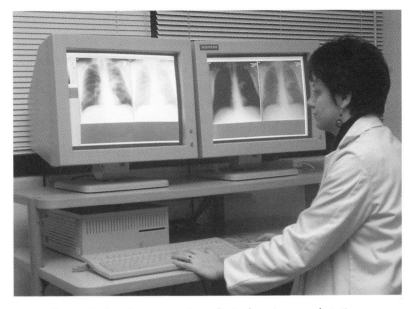

Figure 13.3   A two-monitor clinical review workstation.

information systems (HIS) and radiology information systems (RIS), which do not meet this standard and considerable work has yet to be done with respect to the interfacing of all information systems to ensure the free flow of data in a secure and user-friendly manner. It is essential, therefore, that all future patient information systems embrace these standards so that patient data that may be stored on computers of different types and with different functions is readily accessible at the bedside or in the clinic.

The systems of the future will not carry static images alone, but will need to support a true multimedia environment (text, image, biosignals, voice and colour data). The Commission of the European Community (CEC) has provided funding for several projects in Europe to evaluate the future interface requirements of multimedia developments in medicine. It has also established a project to develop and implement a Good European Health Record (GEHR) system (Lemke, 1993).

CLINICAL ACCEPTANCE OF SOFT-COPY REPORTING

The successful future development of PACSs is dependent upon its acceptance by radiologists and clinicians, which in turn depends upon

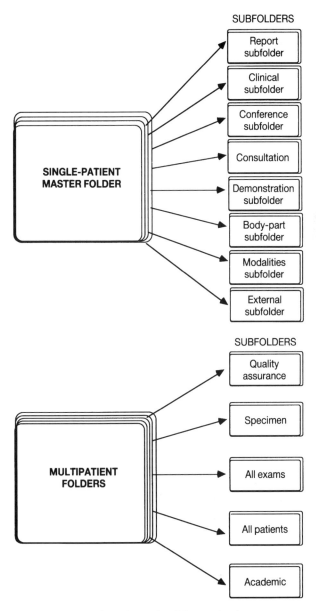

Figure 13.4 Hammersmith Index of Folder-Linked Images (HIFLI). (a) The single-patient master folder concept with the various subfolders contained within it. This allows the user rapid access to the image(s) of interest. (b) The multipatient folder concept which will record images from different patients within a subfolder for such purposes as research and quality assurance.

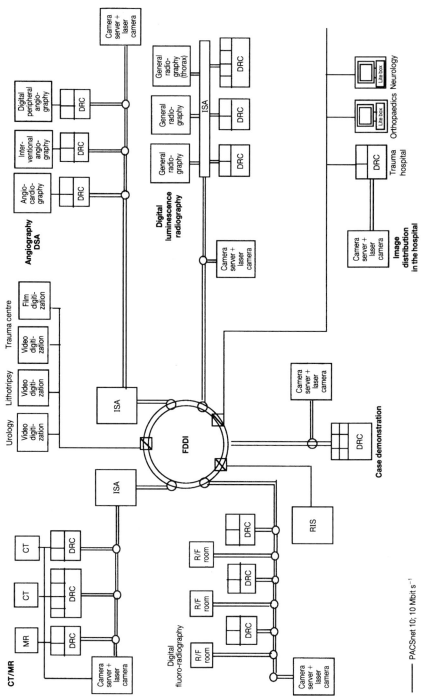

the ease and efficiency with which they can use it. One of the most demanding tasks which will be required of any PACS will be to enable a busy radiologist to undertake a primary reporting session. For 100 years, X-ray film has proved to be a rapid and reliable medium for this task (Foley et al., 1990). Radiological interpretative skills are based, to a considerable extent, on pattern recognition, and many studies have proved that while many films may be displayed during the analysis of a case only a small number are studied in detail (Beend, 1990). According to Strickland and Allison (1995), PACSs must therefore be able to display multiple studies in a manner that allows for their expeditious comparative appraisal, with the minimum amount of image rearrangement.

The facility for image manipulation is an added attraction of soft-copy reporting, since it permits alteration of the grey scale to give both soft-tissue and bone detail, magnification and other diagnosis-enhancing techniques. These image-manipulation capabilities will, however, increase the time taken for reporting, and at present it is estimated that soft-copy reporting will take two or three times longer than conventional reporting if the full diagnostic potential of a PACS is fully to be exploited. Apart from this time consideration, the principal area of concern for radiologists is the inferior spatial resolution of digital images compared with film. Computed radiography (CR) has a standard resolution of 2.5 lines per millimetre compared with 5 lines per millimetre for a standard film–screen combination, and the resolution limitations imposed by the viewing monitor are an additional source of potential image degradation in a PACS. The extent to which these factors are significant in compromising the diagnosis of subtle radiological features has already been the subject of considerable academic interest (MacMalon et al., 1988; Hansell, 1990), but requires further detailed evaluation. So far as we are aware, a study relating to diagnostic efficacy which attempts simultaneously to take into account both the deleterious diagnostic effects of impaired resolution and the beneficial effects of an enhanced image-manipulation capability has yet to be conducted. Whatever the outcome of such a study might be, it is clear that at present the spatial resolution of a video screen is not

Figure 13.5 (opposite)   A schematic representation of the essential components of and their connections within a modular PACS system. FDDI, fibre data distribution interface; ISA, information storage and archiving; DRC, diagnostic reporting consoles; CT, computed tomography; MR, magnetic resonance; DSA, digital subtraction angiography; R/F, radiology fluoroscopy; RIS, radiology information system.

equivalent to that of film; screens are improving rapidly, however, and it is now predicted that not only will relatively low cost 2048^2 display monitors of acceptable quality soon be available but also workstation buses that can move 60 million 32-bit-pixels per second (Beend, 1990). With these significant changes occurring in both the price and technical specifications of modern computer systems, it should not be long before soft-copy reporting of even the subtlest disease changes is feasible. These advances, together with the advantages of image manipulation alluded to above and the facility to gain immediate access to previous images, should guarantee the clinical acceptance of these systems in the near future.

TELERADIOLOGY

The basic concept of a teleradiology system is that two or more sites are connected by communication pathways which enable images and demographic data to be transferred between those sites. The sites concerned may be many miles apart within a country or even in different countries or continents, and the ability to transfer image data between them is principally dependent on the communication systems used. With the expansion of the telecommunication industry there are many choices of interconnection and these include Wide Area Network (WAN), Metropolitan Area Network (MAN), Broadband ISDN telephone lines, and microwave or satellite communications. There are several teleradiology systems in operation throughout the world using different methods of image capture, including film digitization, for example, at the University of California, Los Angeles (Stewart et al., 1992), Madigan Army Medical Centre, Tacona, Washington, and the Direct Digital Capture of Images at the DSAN Hospital, Korea. Such systems are designed to act as an extension to a hospital-based information system, moving the expertise of hospital-lead specialities out into the community.

Exploitation of the potential offered by teleradiology could influence considerably the manner in which imaging is undertaken in the future. It is not outside the realms of possibility that imaging departments and the methods used for referring patients to them will change dramatically over the next 5–7 years, with a large proportion of general radiographic, ultrasonographic and simple contrast studies being carried out in community settings, the images related to these examinations being returned to a central reporting bureau for an expert opinion. General practitioners (GPs) will have the ability, in the future, remotely to request a radiological investigation and to view the resulting images and report on his or her desk-top computer system shortly after completion of the examination.

COST-EFFECTIVENESS

PACS is an expensive tool which, in the present market environment, needs to demonstrate both its clinical usefulness and its economic justification. Information systems have until now been seen as the property of particular departments which have used them to improve their efficiency, enhance their prestige or improve their ability to collect such statistical information as may be desired or required by purchasing authorities, statutory bodies or government departments. They have not in general been seen as mechanisms for effecting changes in diagnostic or management protocols, and their evaluation has been undertaken on a local departmental or hospital basis. PACS and the more sophisticated image-transmission systems now under consideration have much wider implications, however, and the economic studies which are at present under way need to look beyond the limits of the imaging department to ensure that full use is being made of a system's potential, and that the total economic arguments are explored and understood. In Britain, the true economic impact of departmental PACSs is very difficult to establish, because film is much cheaper here than in most other developed countries. For PACSs to be economically viable in this country, it will be necessary for changes to take place in the way hospital clinical staff use the resources at their disposal and just some of the questions we should now be asking ourselves include:

1. Can we use a PACS to improve the methods whereby GPs gain access to a hospital imaging department, and can we modify to advantage the nature and scope of the services those departments offer to the directly referred patient (Gibson et al., 1993)?
2. Do PACSs provide us with an economic argument for moving some imaging facilities into a community-based environment?
3. Can we use hospital facilities in a more appropriate manner, for example streamlining of outpatient appointments and outpatient investigations, streamlining of inpatient investigations, modification of inpatient bed use (Glass, 1992)?
4. Can we use PACSs to establish the correct diagnosis with lower expenditure and fewer investigations (Glass, 1992)?

5. Do PACSs provide us with the opportunity to centralize expertise by enabling experienced staff to supervise examinations undertaken at distant sites?
6. What is the true benefit of our PACS-given ability to undertake telephone and video conferencing between wards and departments or between distant sites?

It will probably take many years to determine whether the PACS can fulfil its clinical potential and prove itself to be financially viable. Attempts to evaluate the benefits and impact of the PACS are clearly fraught with enormous difficulties, and the potential sources of error in such studies are legion; the implications of the PACS for the community, however, in terms of the standards and costs of health care, the planning of community and hospital services, the design of hospital buildings, the distribution of imaging equipment and expertise, and the reorganization of staffing levels and their distribution within the health service are so great that such analyses must be attempted. Very few PACSs are currently large enough to be susceptible to a meaningful assessment of this nature and at Hammersmith Hospital the Health Economics Research Group (HERG) under the direction of Professor Martin Buxton from Brunel University is undertaking a study over a 5-year period funded by the Department of Health. The results are due for publication in 1996.

CONCLUSION

It seems inevitable that PACS and its associated panoply of developments in image manipulation and transmission point the way for the future of medical imaging. Now that the fundamental technical problems seem to have been overcome, it seems certain that the PACS will prove to be to image handling what the telephone proved to be to the spoken word. The PACS is still in its infancy, but its potential is great and the impact it will have on the environment in which we work will be enormous. Imaging departments have been at the forefront of technological development for many years with the introduction of nuclear medicine, computed tomography, magnetic resonance imaging, ultrasound and interventional techniques, but the PACS has the potential to lead us into new and exciting areas and our challenge for the future is to grasp these opportunities and exploit them to the full.

Acknowledgements

The authors would like to thank Professor David Allison, Dr R. A. Reynolds and Dr N. Strickland for their help and support in the writing of this chapter.

References

Allison, D.J., Martin, N.J., Reynolds, R.A. et al. (1994). Clinical aspects of PACS. In Tan, L., Siew, E. (eds) *Proceedings of the 18th International Congress of Radiology*, Singapore, pp 813–819.

Beend, D. (1990) Designing a radiology workstation. A focus on navigation during the interpretation task. *Journal of Digital Imaging* **3**: 152–163.

Bidgood, Jr, W.D., Horil, S.C. (1992) Introduction to the ACR/NEMA DICOM Standard. *Radiographics* **12**: 345–355.

Foley, W.D., Jacobson, D.R., Taylor, A.J. et al. (1990) Display of CT studies on a two screen electronic workstation vs film panel. *Radiology* **174**: 769–773.

Gibson, M.R., Hine, M.R., Shorvan, P.J. (1993) A study of open access ultrasound for GPs. *Proceedings of the Annual Scientific Meeting and Exhibition of the Royal College of Radiologists*, Warwick, p 66. Oxford: Blackwells.

Glass, H. (1992) The impact of PACS on hospital information and practice. *International Journal of Biomedical Computing* **30**: 229–234.

Greenacher, C.F.C., Berthold, S. (1994) Sienet® Installation in routine use: technical commonalties, individual application scenarios, economical facts. *Siemens* **3**: 1.

Hansell, D. (1990) Digital chest radiography: current status. *Clinical Radiology* **41**: 229–231.

Lemke, H.U. (1993) Future directions in electronic image handling. *Investigative Radiology* **28(3)**: S79–81.

MacMalon, H., Metz, C.E., Doi, K. et al. (1988) Digital chest radiography: effect on diagnostic accuracy of hard copy, conventional video and reversed grey scale video display formats. *Radiology* **168(3)**: 669–673.

Stewart, B.K. (1994) Next-generation PACS focus on intelligence. *Diagnostic Imaging International* **10**: 37–39.

Stewart, B.K., Sanuel, J.D., Huang, H.K. et al. (1992) Design of a high-speed, high-resolution teleradiology system. The UCLA PACS research and development programme and related projects. A progress report. Department of Radiological Sciences UCLA CA 90024, USA, pp 100–114. Los Angeles: UCLA.

Strickland, N.H., Allison, D.J. (1995) Default display arrangement of imaging on PACS monitors. *British Journal of Radiology* **68**: 252–260.

14

Trauma Imaging

Miles J. Woodford

INTRODUCTION

Radiography is an essential ingredient in the diagnosis and treatment of trauma. However, its role in the diagnosis of specific injuries is continually being challenged (Baker, 1987) and the number of projections for each radiographic examination is increasingly being evaluated against the ever-rising cost of resources (Bennett et al., 1994), and their place in the management of injuries (Department of Health and Social Security, 1983). Simultaneously, improved levels of care offered to trauma patients by pre-hospital staff are increasing the numbers of patients with severe injuries who are presenting to accident and emergency (A&E) departments. High-quality radiographs are, nevertheless, expected, irrespective of the condition of the patient.

LITERATURE

A literature search failed to find references to recent changes in trauma radiography. Indeed, the search highlighted the lack of radiographic publications in the entire field of trauma.

There were many references to the radiology of trauma (Hodgkinson et al., 1993), and each of these obliquely referred to the radiographic examinations. The emphasis was on the radiological evidence that may be discernible (Shaffer and Doris, 1981), and the pitfalls associated with a failure to demonstrate or perceive information

(Vandermark, 1990). Similarly, there are references to the efficacy of particular radiographic protocols in the evaluation of specific injuries, for example cervical spine injury (Woodray and Lee, 1993), head injury (South East Thames Regional Health Authority, 1989) and the use of ultrasound in blunt abdominal trauma.

Recent reports highlight the need for increased resources for trauma victims, balancing the significant costs of accidents against the evaluation of outcomes following major trauma. The implications or costs of accidents include those to:

1. Society in general.
2. The individual and his or her family.
3. The National Health Service (NHS).

Accidents primarily affect people in the younger age groups, causing death or disability to people who are, commonly, on the threshold of adult life and, in many cases, with young families. The cost of a father, son, sister, husband or wife are, of course, incalculable. However, whilst there is great sorrow on reading of the death of an accident victim in the local paper, the seriously injured are largely forgotten and the major problems they face usually ignored. Many will be permanently disabled and most face a stiff battle if they are to regain their previous place in society. It is estimated that for every death caused by road accidents there are likely to be two or three permanently disabled victims and many more who are temporarily disabled (Harris et al., 1989). The public is not alone in finding it easy to count the number of deaths, but difficult to comprehend how much disability and hardship are caused by accidents. Deaths, whilst concrete and countable, are but the tip of the iceberg. The difficulty is in measuring the costs, in all senses, of the large numbers of people who become disabled as a result of road accidents.

Research in this country and abroad, mainly in the USA where it provided the rationale for trauma-centre development, has suggested that of early deaths due to brain injury, thoracic trauma or severe haemorrhage, up to 30% were avoidable given proper management of the airway plus appropriate and timely management of bleeding (Baker, 1987) . Despite some advances, the present systems of care for trauma victims in the UK remain poor (Waters, 1992). The ideal trauma care system is undoubtedly the so-called 'trauma centre' where those suffering major trauma are assessed and treated by senior staff in all of the relevant major specialities. These doctors are dedicated to the management of trauma and are available immediately, 24 hours a day. Unfortunately, such centres are horrendously expensive to run and, even in the USA which has a much larger trauma load, the costs of such units are being questioned.

At the same time, the outcome in terms of survival of major trauma patients is also being audited according to the TRISS method (Boyd et al., 1987). This method combines assessment of the anatomical injury (Injury Severity Score (ISS)) (Baker et al., 1974) and the physiological injury (Revised Trauma Score (RTS)), and has been shown to provide a better than 95% prediction of outcome of major injury in terms of survival for any given institution. Deviations can be investigated with a view to prevention when there is unexpected death, or consolidation when there is unexpected survival (Marmaris and Brooks, 1990), and a comparison of performances in trauma care amongst institutions can be made (Bennett et al., 1994).

CHANGES IN TRAUMA CARE

The introduction of a primary radiographic survey as part of an advanced trauma life support (ATLS) procedure has focused attention on an immediate evaluation of the patient from a clinical examination, together with radiographs of the lateral cervical spine, the chest and the pelvis (Hodgkinson et al., 1993). The emphasis on early homeostasis with immediate respiratory treatment may require repeated chest radiography of consistent standards for strict comparison and, thereby, evaluation of the treatment.

The secondary (full) survey follows stabilization of the patient, and may occur in the resuscitation room, the radiographic department, or the operating theatre. The time interval between the primary survey and removal of the patient to the operating theatre may be as little as 20 minutes. It is during this period of secondary survey that a full radiographic examination will be made. This will complete the primary survey of the cervical spine and other body areas, and may also include arteriography, ultrasound and image intensification.

The Radiographic Service

The selection of a suitable film–screen combination will produce a system with wide photographic latitude and high speed. The latitude is essential to produce chest and cervical spine images which demonstrate both bony- and soft-tissue information. The high speed reduces the risk of blurring from uncontrolled patient movements whilst enabling lower exposures, so maintaining low doses for staff who are necessarily close to the patient during radiographic examinations.

X-ray equipment may be a mobile unit or a ceiling-suspended unit providing consistent high-powered exposure outputs coupled with excellent tube-head manoeuvrability.

Radiographers will be expected to have a wide range of skills in producing high-quality images, regardless of the circumstances, often during the night-time, and, therefore, without the full back-up of the radiology department. Radiography managers, responsible for providing an out-of-hours service may limit the on-call rota to junior staff, with senior members allocated to second on-call. It is not uncommon for the least experienced members of staff to be responsible for producing images under the most difficult of conditions. More senior members of staff may perform the secondary radiographic surveys over long periods of time, so contributing to the high cost of trauma care, an important issue in the debate about the future of specialist trauma centres.

In centres that have introduced trauma teams, the radiographer may be included in the trauma team and will be expected to be available with the other members of the team. Such radiographers may find themselves trained and encouraged to play an active role in the reception of the trauma victim. In these circumstances, it is common for radiographers to be expected to help with the interpretation of images, and with the selection of appropriate complementary projections to complete the diagnosis.

Radiography of the Cervical Spine

Many centres rely on a horizontal ray lateral (HRL) projection as the mainstay of the radiographic evaluation of cervical spine trauma. Indeed, it is the sole projection of the cervical spine within the primary survey in the ATLS procedure. The value of this projection is a compound of its radiographic ease, of not incurring movement of the patient, and of its positive pick-up rate of 75%. However, it has limitations.

The projection must include all seven cervical vertebrae and the cervical–thoracic junction. The mandible should not be superimposed on the anterior portion of the body of the second cervical vertebra, and both soft tissue and bony information needs to demonstrated. Modern radiographic equipment and a suitable film–screen combination will employ short exposure times to produce radiographs displaying wide photographic latitude and the required information.

The difficulty of demonstrating the cervical–thoracic junction is well known, but the importance of doing so cannot be overemphasized. A radiographic technique using arm traction applied by experienced and trained personnel, together with suspended expiration, will help to display the junction.

Failure to demonstrate the junction will result in the need to undertake a 'swimmer projection', during which one arm is raised above the head. In this procedure, the grid cassette is placed in the axilla of the raised arm, and the opposite arm is positioned alongside the patient. The central ray is directed toward the acromioclavicular joint and toward the grid cassette at 90° to the long axis of the spine. The projection will demonstrate vertebral alignment and the airway and, from the position of the disc spaces, vertebral height. It is an extremely difficult projection to carry out on an unconscious patient and is impossible in patients with upper extremity injuries. It is almost completely contraindicated in patients with signs of cervical cord injury.

The standard horizontal ray lateral projection of the cervical vertebrae has been shown to produce a false-negative rate of 25% (Shaffer and Doris, 1981) and it must be emphasized that the levels of patient care must not be lowered when there are no positive radiographic findings. The cervical collar must remain in situ until the patient is stabilized fully.

Chest Injuries and Radiography

There are three main mechanisms of chest trauma: low-velocity impact, high-velocity impact, and crush injury.

Low-velocity impacts from direct blows to the chest wall result in unilateral rib fractures, or sternal fractures, and can be associated with pulmonary and cardiac contusion. The rib fractures are best diagnosed clinically and a chest radiograph will determine the presence or absence of associated intrathoracic injuries.

High-velocity impacts from deceleration effects in road traffic accidents result in bilateral rib fractures, or sternal fractures, and can be associated with a ruptured aorta, diaphragm or bronchus, or with cardiac contusion.

Crush injuries result in: bilateral rib fractures, with or without a flail segment; ipsilateral rib fractures, with or without a flail segment; or, possibly, contralateral rib fractures. These can be associated with a ruptured bronchus, or with cardiac or pulmonary contusion. A flail segment may be associated with serious intrathoracic injury, especially pulmonary contusion, and may progress to respiratory failure.

Chest radiography is a great asset in the evaluation of all the above conditions but, ideally, must demonstrate mediastinal and peripheral lung information in a single radiograph. The radiographic technique of choice, therefore, involves selection of a high peak kilovoltage, the use of a secondary radiation grid and a suitable latitude film–screen combination.

Pelvis

There are three main mechanisms of pelvic trauma: anteroposterior compression, lateral compression and vertical shear force. In under 25% of cases, there may be a combination of two of these mechanisms.

Anteroposterior compression may disrupt the pubic symphysis, may fracture the pubic rami, and may disrupt the ligaments associated with the sacroiliac joints. An anteroposterior force may also push the flexed femur posteriorly, fracturing the posterior margin of the acetabulum. Lateral compression may cause a horizontal fracture through the pubic symphysis and may centrally dislocate the hip, while vertical shearing tears the sacroiliac ligaments and the pubic symphysis ligaments, and is associated with pelvic instability and vascular damage.

An anteroposterior radiograph of the pelvis will be sufficiently diagnostic in 94% of all cases of pelvic injury.

CONCLUSION

The functions of A&E departments are being measured, using the TRISS method (Marmaris and Brooks, 1990), to focus attention on results and outcomes. The success of improvements in trauma management are financially assessed and compared with the costs. The costs of radiography are considerable.

The choice of no radiographic procedure, plain skull radiography or computed tomography for the head-injured patient typifies the problems faced by the radiographer in the A&E department.

Many recent studies (Department of Health and Social Security, 1983; Bennett et al., 1994) suggest that only patients with specific neurological symptoms should be investigated radiographically, using computed tomography. However, plain film radiography of the skull for minor head injuries remains prevalent.

Regional radiographic guidelines (South East Thames Regional Health Authority, 1989) have managed to reduce the number of patients receiving plain-film radiography without altering the success of their management. However, within these guidelines, there is the facility for the development of local modifications, tailored to individual requirements and resources. There are still pressures from A&E clinicians to carry out plain-film skull radiography for medico-legal reasons, and to satisfy patients' expectations, regardless of clinical judgement.

None of these decisions are made by radiographers, and although trauma radiography is a large percentage of a radiography department's workload, decisions on its relevance remain the curious province of A&E consultants. Radiologists, and especially radiographers, and their respective professional bodies have little or no long-term effect on these decisions.

References

Baker, S.P. (1987) Injuries: the neglected epidemic. Stone Lecture 1985. America Trauma Society Meeting. *Journal of Trauma* **27:** 343–348.

Baker, S.P., O'Neill, B., Haddon, W.J. et al. (1974) The Injury Severity Score: a method for describing patients with multiple injuries and evaluating trauma care. *Journal of Trauma* **14:** 187–196.

Bennett, J., Penz-Avila, C.A., Wallace, S.A. et al. (1994) Head injuries in the A/E department: are we using resources effectively? *Journal of A/E Medicine* **11:** 25–31.

Boyd, C.R., Tolson, M.A., Copes, W.S. (1987) Evaluating trauma care: the TRISS method. *Journal of Trauma* **27:** 370–378.

Department of Health and Social Security (1983) The management of acute head injury. *Harrogate Seminar Report No. 8.* DHSS: London.

Harris, B.H., Schwaitzberg, S.D., Seman, T.M. et al. (1989) The hidden morbidity of paediatric trauma. *Journal of Paediatric Surgery* **24:** 103–105.

Hodgkinson, D.W., O'Driscoll, B.R., Driscoll, P.A. et al. (1993) ABC of emergency radiographs – II. *British Medical Journal* **307:** 1273–1277.

Marmaris, C., Brooks, S.C. (1990) Monitoring progress in major trauma care using TRISS. *Archives of Emergency Medicine* **7:** 169–171.

Royal College of Radiologists Working Party. (1983) Patient selection for skull radiology in uncomplicated head injury. *Lancet* **115:** 8.

Shaffer, M.A., Doris, P.E. (1981) Limitations of the cross table lateral view in detecting cervical spine injuries: a retrospective analysis. *Annals of Emergency Medicine* **10:** 508.

South East Thames Regional Health Authority (1989) *A Regional Policy. Care of Patients with Acute Head Injury in District General Hospitals.* South East Thames RHA: Bexhill-on-Sea.

Vandermark, R.M. (1990) Radiology of the cervical spine in trauma patients. Practice, pitfalls and recommendations for improving efficiency and communications. *American Journal of Roentgenology* **155:** 465.

Waters, E. (1992) Road traffic accidents. *Salisbury Medical Bulletin* **75:** 15–20.

Woodray, J.H., Lee, C. (1993) Limitations of cervical radiography in the evaluation of acute cervical trauma. *Journal of Trauma* **34:** 32–39.

15

The Value of the 18-Week Scan in the Second Trimester of Pregnancy

Josephine Swallow

INTRODUCTION

Almost all hospitals in the UK now offer a routine ultrasound scan to all patients at 18–20 weeks gestation. Figure 15.1 illustrates a typical image obtained during such a scan.

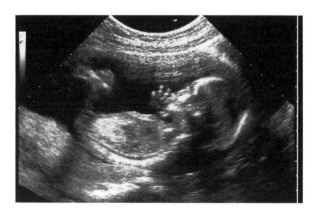

Figure 15.1 Typical image obtained during an 18-week scan.

The reasons for undertaking this scan are:

1. To establish the viability and maturity of the fetus.
2. To exclude major structural abnormalities.
3. To diagnose multiple pregnancy.
4. To develop a bond between parents and fetus.

When the mother books into the antenatal clinic, a careful obstetric history is recorded which often provides the key to an accurate sonographic diagnosis. During the scan the sonographer has the opportunity to listen to the patient's complaints of illness through pregnancy and, on some occasions, may obtain information that the patient has not shared with the referring clinician.

Before the value of the 18-week scan in the second trimester can be discussed the following should be explained:

1. What is an 18-week anomaly scan?
2. What results may be obtained from it?
3. How is it performed?

THE 18-WEEK ANOMALY SCAN

Routine obstetric scanning at 18–20 weeks was introduced into the UK in the early 1980s and is recommended by the Royal College of Obstetricians and Gynaecologists (1984). This is the optimum time during gestation for visualization of fetal anatomy. Successful ultrasound diagnosis lies in the ability to obtain detailed images in which a maximum of anatomical information is presented. The examiner must be able to recognize normal sonographic appearances and to demonstrate them accurately.

Routine ultrasound scanning is effective in the detection of fetal abnormalities (Chitty et al., 1991) and must be performed by professionally trained and highly skilled sonologists/sonographers. Sensitivities of 60.7% to 74.4% and specificities of 99% for the detection of all structural malformations have been reported from two centres in the UK (Chitty, 1994). Serious or lethal abnormalities give a higher sensitivity level of 72–83%.

INFORMATION AVAILABLE FROM AN 18-WEEK SCAN

Abnormalities are present in 14% of newborn infants and major abnormalities are present in 2–5% of fetuses. These account for 20–30% of prenatal deaths. Congenital anomalies consist of departures from the normal anatomical architecture of organs or systems and may be split into two groups.

1. *Major*: these are anomalies with medical, surgical or cosmetic importance, with impacts on morbidity and mortality.
2. *Minor*: these anomalies do not have serious medical or surgical significance and do not affect normal life expectancy.

It is critical that when one abnormality has been detected, others should be searched for, as there is often more than one major abnormality present. Abnormality detection is analysed by organ system:

1. Central nervous system.
2. Cardiac system.
3. Lungs and diaphragm.
4. Gastrointestinal system.
5. Renal system.
6. Skeletal system.

Table 15.1 demonstrates the types of abnormalities routinely detected.

Table 15.1   Abnormalities detected from an 18–20 week scan

Craniospinal defects	*Gastrointestinal anomalies*	*Skeletal anomalies*
Anencephaly	Omphocele	Achondrogenesis
Spina bifida	Gastroschisis	Achondroplasia
Encephalocele	Umbilical hernia	Amelia
Iniencephaly	Diaphragmatic hernia	Phocomelia
Holoprosencephaly	Duodenal atresia	Limb reduction deformity
Hydranencephaly	Jejunal atresia	Absent radius or ulna
Microcephaly	Meconium peritonitis	Diastrophic dwarf
Sacral agenesis	Chronic obstruction	Thanatophoric dwarf
Absent cerebellum		Osteogenesis imperfecta
Dandy–Walker syndrome	*Urinary tract anomalies*	Facial defects
Joubert's syndrome	Obstructive uropathy	
Porencephalic cysts	Infantile polycystic	*Cadiac anomalies*
Macrocephaly	disease	Atrial septal defects
	Meckel's syndrome	Ventricular septal defects
Fetal tumours	Renal agenesis	Mitral atresia
Cystic hygroma	Renal dysplasia	Ebstein's anomaly
Neuroblastoma	Unilateral and bilateral	Hypoplastic left heart
Sacral teratoma	renal cysts	Non-immune hydrops
	Cloacal extrophy	
	Nephroblastoma	

Effective therapy should be available for any problems detected. Medical and surgical possibilities exist for many congenital anomalies. An early diagnosis may be followed by karyotyping or possible prenatal therapy. If an abnormality is not treatable and is incompatible with life, a termination of the pregnancy may be offered. The mother should be transferred to a special-care facility centre for delivery of an abnormal fetus so that immediate optimum care may be given.

An ultrasound scan also provides information on gestational age, viability and the number of fetuses present. Placental position and liquor volume are also examined. The majority of pregnant women in the UK now receive at least one ultrasound scan, which should be performed at the optimum time of 18–20 weeks gestation.

The issue for the patient is one of information and choice. The 18-week scan should be fully explained to the patient and the reasons for the scan given. The patient then has a choice as to whether or not she undertakes to have the scan. In particular, she should be informed that an abnormality, either major or minor, may be detected. This may require her to make a choice about the future of her child. It is now possible to correct certain conditions in utero, and decisions involving the parents and specialists may be needed.

PARAMETERS AND TECHNIQUE OF AN 18-WEEK SCAN

Measurements

The following measurements should be performed to establish gestational age and exclude abnormality:

1. Biparietal diameter (BPD).
2. Head circumference.
3. Anterior and posterior ventricular horns (see Figure 15.2).
4. Cerebral hemisphere.
5. Femur length (see Figure 15.3).
6. Nuchal-fold thickness, a soft marker (see Figure 15.4).

Identification

The following structures must be identified:

1. Cerebellum.
2. Spine in longitudinal and transverse sections.

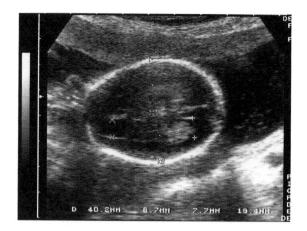

Figure 15.2   Anterior and posterior horns of the lateral ventricles.

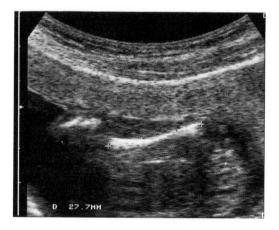

Figure 15.3   Femur length.

3. Heart in the four-chamber view, and the heart beat.
4. Chest, diaphragm and stomach, which should be seen below the diaphragm on the left.
5. Abdominal wall and cord insertion; three vessels should be visualized in the cord (see Figure 15.5).
6. Kidneys and bladder should be present and normal in size.
7. Four limbs.

Other structures may also be identified in a more detailed scan. These include: the orbits; the facial bones; lips and hard palate; liver;

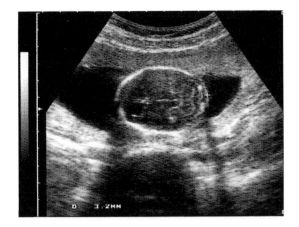

Figure 15.4   Nuchal-fold thickness.

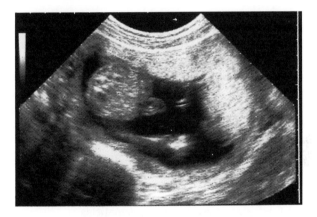

Figure 15.5   Cord insertion.

detailed cardiac scan; and digits. Finally, assessment of the amniotic fluid and the placental site is made.

More recently, the presence of 'soft markers' has drawn attention to the possibility of chromosomal aberrations. The risk of a chromosomal abnormality from a single soft marker is extremely low, but combinations of markers increase the risk and karyotyping should be offered if two or more soft markers are present. The most common soft markers are:

1. Choroid plexus cysts.
2. Nuchal fat pad in excess of 6 mm.

3. Echogenic focus in left and right ventricles of heart.
4. 'Bright' (echo-rich) bowel.
5. Dilated renal pelves with pelvic widths greater than 4 mm.

Such markers are most commonly associated with trisomy 21, 18 and 13 syndromes.

ULTRASOUND APPEARANCES OF FETAL ABNORMALITIES

Craniospinal Abnormalities

Approximately 50–65% of all neural tube defects are anencephaly. This is the easiest craniospinal abnormality to diagnose and is the most gross form of open neural tube defect, being incompatible with life.

Spina bifida, both open and closed lesions, is a failure of one or more of the vertebral arches to fuse. The meninges may herniate through the bony defect, forming a soft tissue mass of variable size. This is a meningocele if it contains no nervous tissue, and a meningomyelocele if it contains nervous tissue. Of all spina bifida lesions, 90% are lumbar, 6% are thoracic and 3% are cervical lesions. The ultrasonic appearance of a 'lemon-shaped' head is diagnostic of a neural tube defect. The dilated ventricles are obvious and the cerebellum appears banana-shaped rather than dumb-bell-shaped. There is widening of the spine in the anteroposterior view and a cup-shaped appearance in the transverse view.

Abdomen and Gastrointestinal Tract Abnormalities

Omphocele

This is a mass, or herniation, with a membranous covering, arising from the fetal abdomen. The mass contains loops of bowel and/or liver, spleen and pancreas. The umbilical cord is inserted into the apex of the mass. There is a high incidence (of the order of 30–60%) of associated malformations and with chromosome abnormalities.

Eventration

This is a special form of omphocele in which the abdominal contents herniate through a large central abdominal wall defect and are in direct contact with the chorion of the placenta. It is covered only by a short piece of umbilical cord.

Gastroschisis

The defect is on the right abdominal wall, lateral and inferior to the umbilicus. The cord is separate. Bowel loops are seen floating in the amniotic fluid and are not covered by a membrane. Gastroschisis is usually an isolated defect.

Upper abdomen

Duodenal atresia is recognized by a 'double-bubble' sign. One bubble represents the overdistended stomach and the other bubble is the fluid-filled segment of duodenum between the pylorus and the stenosis. It may be associated with chromosomal abnormalities. Jejunal atresia is quite rare and gives a triple-bubble sign.

Diaphragmatic hernia is demonstrated by fluid-filled spaces in the chest and is usually left-sided. This is due to stomach and bowel herniating into the chest. Pulmonary hypoplasia may result.

Urinary Tract Abnormalities

The commonest reason for referral is oligohydramnios, which holds a very poor prognosis and which may be due to renal agenesis or to very severe growth retardation. If, however, one kidney is functioning normally, the prognosis is good. In Potter's syndrome there is a complete absence of the kidneys and the resultant oligohydramnios makes the fetus very difficult to examine ultrasonically.

Obstructive uropathies are a range of conditions in which there is an obstruction in some part of the urinary tract. In pelvi-ureteric obstruction there is a dilated renal pelvis and well-preserved renal cortex. There is good renal function, adequate amniotic fluid and good fetal bladder filling. Posterior urethral valves show a distended bladder, which can be treated with a bladder shunt before any cortical damage has been done to the kidney.

Hydrops Fetalis

Ultrasonically, there is excessive fluid accumulation in the body cavities and/or soft tissue oedema. This may be caused by rhesus isoimmunization, but as rhesus disease is now rare it is more commonly of the non-hydrops type for which there are a number of causes.

ADVANTAGES OF THE 18-WEEK SCAN

The ultrasound scan provides an opportunity for the parents and other children to 'bond' to the new baby. Most experiences are happy and parents leave (usually with a picture) feeling confident that their new baby is alive and structurally normal. This must not be underestimated, particularly when parents have experienced a previous miscarriage or fetal abnormality.

The correction of inaccurate dating of the pregnancy and the early diagnosis of multiple gestations is an advantage when planning delivery time, mode of delivery and making domestic arrangements.

The advantages of the 18-week scan from an economic standpoint are that early diagnosis of severely disabling abnormalities and the offer of selective termination, when appropriate, could be cost-effective in the long term. Early recognition and treatment may be highly cost-effective if it prevents handicap from chronic disease. Ultrasound is relatively inexpensive compared to other imaging modalities and a machine capable of producing a high-resolution image may be purchased for approximately £20 000.

Detection of an abnormality allows the parents to make a choice, after expert counselling, regarding the continuation of the pregnancy. If the parents elect to continue with the pregnancy despite the outcome being extremely poor, they can be given full support during the pregnancy. The fetus can be delivered where there are appropriate neonatal facilities and an appropriate method of delivery can be discussed beforehand. For example, a gastroschisis can be successfully repaired at a recognized centre.

Even when problems are identified, studies suggest that couples still appreciate that they were able to participate in the scan and see the fetus. If the condition is lethal, a photograph offered at an appropriate time, and with sensitivity, often helps the grieving process. It also gives parents time to prepare for the death of their baby if they elect to continue with the pregnancy to its natural conclusion.

The presence of minor anomalies, for example cleft lip, gives the parents time to prepare themselves for the birth and to meet other parents who have had infants with similar conditions. Support groups are available for parents facing such difficulties.

Some parents are only prepared to accept a 'perfect' baby and a minor abnormality such as a cleft lip or a shortened limb may be considered by them to be ample justification to seek a termination of pregnancy. This raises a host of moral and ethical issues: 'The failure of society to achieve emotional resolution and political clarity regarding the sanctity of life with regard to selective fetal termination has created a tenuous legal and moral climate' (Weiss, 1985). If a patient elects to terminate her pregnancy, the sonographer should avoid judging her morally, realizing that the patient and her physicians have based their decisions on multiple factors, some of which may be unknown to the sonographer. It is not in the sonographer's brief to withhold information regarding minor abnormalities in order to avoid these issues.

If an abnormality is present, fetal karyotyping may be discussed. If the karyotype is abnormal further counselling should take place with the geneticist and the obstetrician, so that an informed decision can be made by the parents as to whether the pregnancy should continue. Again the presence of two or more 'soft markers', as previously described, may influence the parents to accept karyotyping. A surgically correctable abnormality with normal karyotyping may persuade the parents to continue with the pregnancy. Once the parents elect to continue, they should be given as much support as possible and, at the earliest opportunity, meet the team that will care for their infant.

There are no confirmed adverse effects of diagnostic ultrasound used in vivo by suitably qualified sonographers. These are people who are aware of the studies on adverse and bio-effects and use ultrasound prudently following the 'as low as is reasonably achievable' (ALARA) principle. There is growing awareness of acoustic exposures, and all manufacturers should produce data relating to equipment output, intensity and pressure amplitude. Manufacturers are in the process of implementing on-screen, real-time displays of the acoustic power of their machines. All equipment should be checked regularly by a medical physicist. The knowledge and the skill of the user are the major determinants of the risk–benefit implications, and an unrealistic emphasis on the safety of ultrasound energy may discourage the appropriate use of ultrasound.

POSSIBLE DISADVANTAGES OF THE 18-WEEK SCAN

If parents are not informed before the scan that an anomaly may be found, the effect on them may be devastating if they had high expectations of a happy, largely social, scan.

Two recent publications, including the RADIUS report from North America (Ednigman et al., 1993) failed to demonstrate any significant benefit from ultrasound. There were no significant differences in the rate of adverse perinatal outcome in terms of fetal or neonatal death, or substantial neonatal morbidity. The RADIUS study reported much lower rates of detection of abnormalities than the studies described recently in the UK (Shirley et al., 1992; Chitty et al., 1994). However, it used a selected population rather than one which reflects the general population.

Anxiety levels may be raised if the scan proves to be technically difficult, for example if the mother is large or if the fetus is in a difficult position. The mother may then be asked to return for a repeat scan at a later date. Much anxiety can also be caused by the present of 'soft markers'. Even after careful counselling, the doubt that there may be an abnormality remains with the parents until the infant is born. The uncertainty of the relevance of these 'soft markers' in relation to chromosome abnormalities causes great concern, and inappropriate counselling may also add to the anxiety of parents.

When an abnormality is detected and the parents make a decision to elect for a termination, they may be totally unprepared for the grief process which will inevitably follow. They may experience feelings of guilt for ending a much-wanted pregnancy which may outweigh the alternative decision of 'leaving things to nature' and coping with a stillbirth or neonatal death.

The value of treating fetuses in utero is also in question, particularly for renal obstruction and hydrocephalus. In the case of hydrocephalus it has been concluded that in utero shunting carries no benefit and there is now an international moratorium on fetal intervention for hydrocephalus.

Many papers have been produced recently on the possible adverse effects of ultrasound, which may make parents worry as to any possible effect ultrasound could have on their baby. Papers include studies of a higher incidence of growth retardation in pregnancies exposed to repeated ultrasound scans and the observation of a greater incidence of left-handedness in infants (Newham et al., 1993; Salveson et al., 1993). These observed results may, however, be due to chance and more rigorous research is required.

CONCLUSION

The preceding sections have raised arguments both for and against the routine 18-week obstetric ultrasound scan. However, for many parents and obstetricians the benefits far outweigh the disadvantages. Key benefits are:

1. That the parents are given the opportunity to bond with their baby.
2. Information can be obtained to determine whether the fetus is anatomically normal.
3. Multiple pregnancy can be excluded, or, alternatively, parents can prepare for a multiple birth.
4. The gestational age of the fetus can be established.

If the following guidelines are observed, routine scanning should continue to be relatively safe, efficient and cost-effective:

1. Standardization of the training of sonographers.
2. Operators to be suitably qualified and facilities available for their continuing education.
3. Monitoring and audit of staff performance.
4. Available equipment should be able to produce high-quality images.

References

Chitty, L.S. (1994) Controversies in ultrasound. *British Medical Ultrasound Society Bulletin* **Feb.:** 31–32.

Chitty, L.S., Hunt, G.H., Moore, J. (1991) Effectiveness of routine ultrasonography in detecting fetal structural abnormalities in low risk population. *British Medical Journal* **303:** 1665–1669.

Ednigman, B.G., Crane, J.P., Frigoletto F.D. et al. (1993) Effect of prenatal ultrasound screening on perinatal outcome. *New England Journal of Medicine* **329:** 821–827.

Newham, J.P., Evans, S.F., Michael, C.A. et al. (1993) Effects of frequent ultrasound during pregnancy. A randomised control trial. *Lancet* **342:** 887–891.

Royal College of Obstetricians and Gynaecologists Working Party (1984) *Working Party Report on Routine Ultrasound Examinations in Pregnancy* London: RCOG.

Salveson, K.A., Vatten, L.J., Eik-Nes, S.H., et al. (1993) Routine ultrasonography in utero and subsequent handedness and neurological developments. *British Medical Journal* **307:** 159–164.

Shirley, I.M., Bottomley, F., Robinson, V.P. (1992) Routine radiography screening for fetal abnormality by ultrasound in an unselected low risk population. *British Journal of Radiology* **65:** 564–569.

16

Intraoperative Ultrasound in Hepatic Resection

Jane A. Bates and Rose Marie Conlon

INTRODUCTION

Intraoperative ultrasound (IOUS) was first used in the early 1960s. The advantages of IOUS have been recognized for many years. The limitation of acoustic attenuation through subcutaneous tissue or bone can be eliminated, allowing direct contact with an organ and enabling the use of a high-frequency transducer. It is inexpensive and safe, and there are no recorded complications (e.g. hepatic injury or infection) due to its use.

Until recently, the technique was confined to specialized centres, but increasing demand over a wide variety of applications has allowed IOUS to develop rapidly, with more readily available dedicated equipment and operator expertise. The applications of IOUS are varied, including neurosurgical procedures for precise localization of lesions for biopsy and surgery and vascular procedures, in which IOUS can demonstrate atheroma, vessel wall anatomy and patency after reconstructive surgery. In the abdomen, IOUS has been used for some years to localize renal calculi prior to their removal, and biliary calculi, particularly those in the distal common bile duct. More recently, IOUS has become recognized as a useful tool in the examination of the pancreas for small tumours and inflammatory lesions. It is also used in the staging of secondary ovarian tumours and in the surgical management of thyroid and parathyroid glands.

BACKGROUND

The recent reported success of surgical liver resection for hepatic metastases has prompted wider interest in IOUS. The most common cause for referral for liver resection is colorectal carcinoma, in which over 20% of patients have liver metastases at the time of laparotomy (Freeny and Marks, 1986). Unlike some primary carcinomas, in which metastatic spread to the liver makes further therapy of no benefit, a potential cure is possible with colorectal carcinoma, depending on the number and position of hepatic secondary deposits. Liver metastases are the cause of death in 60–70% of patients with colorectal carcinoma (Russo and Sparacino, 1989). Patients with hepatic metastases from colorectal carcinoma do not usually survive beyond 12 months if untreated, with an average survival period of 8 months (Bengmark and Hafstrom, 1978). However, a 5-year survival rate has been reported in 20–40% of patients after liver resection for three or fewer metastases (Adson et al., 1984; Sugarbaker and Kemeny, 1988). This figure could, potentially, be improved with better patient selection and preoperative staging. Liver resections are also carried out for cholangiocarcinoma, hepatoma and, less frequently, for trauma.

DIAGNOSIS AND STAGING

The management of colorectal carcinoma depends largely upon the number and extent of liver metastases present. Accurate assessment of the number, size and position of deposits is essential, and various preoperative imaging techniques are employed, including computed tomography (CT), transabdominal ultrasound and magnetic resonance imaging (MRI). In our establishment elective patients undergo a vigorous preoperative work-up:

1. Carcinoembryonic antigen (CEA) levels.
2. Ultrasound scan.
3. MRI of the liver.
4. CT of the chest, abdomen and pelvis.
5. Exercise ECG.
6. Lung function.

It is from this preoperative assessment that a patient is deemed suitable for surgical resection or is referred for chemotherapy.

An uncomplicated liver resection takes approximately 3–4 hours, but frequently because of the findings during surgery the planned resection is altered and the operation may last for up to 10 hours. For example, in a recent case, tumour was found to be infiltrating the lateral border of the right kidney (undetected preoperatively) and a partial nephrectomy was necessary.

Patients are usually encephalopathic for a few days postoperatively and this has to be monitored carefully. Long-term postoperative follow-up at our hospital involves:

1. CEA at 3, 6, 12 months and annually for 5 years.
2. CT of the liver at 3 months.
3. CT of the chest, abdomen and pelvis, at 12 months.
4. Ultrasound follow-up annually for 5 years.

A significant contribution to failure of hepatic resection is the inability of conventional preoperative staging to detect some small metastases, resulting in recurrence of the disease. Detection rates for hepatic metastases tend to be somewhat institution-specific, depending on techniques and equipment. CT sensitivities as low as 38% have been reported (Heiken et al., 1989), but this can be improved by using bolus-contrast-delayed CT. CT with arterial portography would seem to give the best results (up to 81%) (Heiken et al., 1989), but this is highly invasive, time-consuming and suffers from a significant false-positive rate in some series. Most recent series quote sensitivities of between 47% and 65% for CT (Machi et al., 1991; Stewart et al., 1993).

MRI is now generally reported to surpass the sensitivity of CT, and has certainly become more readily available in recent years. The detection rate is difficult to estimate without suitable follow-up, but a recent series detected 281 lesions using a combination of sequences, as opposed to 220 with CT (Semelka et al., 1992). Some small lesions are still known to go undetected, and the sensitivity is probably of the order of 90%.

Palpation of the liver at surgery is known to exceed the sensitivities of most preoperative imaging modalities (Machi et al., 1991; Stewart et al., 1993; Knol et al., 1993), detecting up to 82% of lesions, but small, deep metastases cannot be palpated, particularly in the posterior aspect of the right lobe. Also, adhesions may prevent accurate palpation by the surgeon. IOUS detects more hepatic metastases than any preoperative imaging technique currently available, with sensitivities of 82–97.8% (Machi et al., 1987, 1991; Stewart et al., 1993; Knol et al., 1993), but tends to miss superficial lesions, due to poor visualization immediately adjacent to the transducer face. This does not present a clinical problem, however, as such lesions are readily visualized and palpated. In the most recently published series (Kane et al., 1994) of 154 lesions, 150 were detected by IOUS and three of the four remaining ones were readily detectable by surgical palpation, giving a sensitivity of 99.4% for these combined techniques, which far exceeds that of preoperative imaging. Lesions of 5 mm in diameter and less are now regularly seen with IOUS.

EQUIPMENT

The vast choice of scanning equipment includes dedicated intraoperative machines with sterilizable probes and surfaces. The equipment of choice must be easily portable and be able to be cleaned thoroughly, but we have not found it necessary to use a dedicated intraoperative machine in our institution. Indeed, the small, relatively cheap, portable scanner in use has several advantages, including simplicity of controls.

The obvious priority is for a high-resolution image. The design and frequency of the transducer is, of course, a matter of individual choice. In our experience a linear T-shaped probe (Figure 16.1) allows by far the best image quality, particularly in the near field, together with ease of use and image interpretation. This design of probe is very useful in limited spaces where access is difficult, for example around the lateral and superior margins of the liver. Other probe designs on the market include a side-firing I-shaped linear array, which affords the same image quality but requires the operator to scan with the probe along the index finger in order to maintain surface contact. This is difficult, particularly at the lower edge of the liver. Some operators recommend

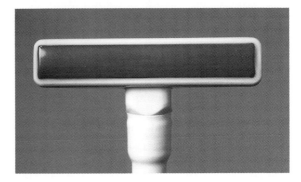

Figure 16.1   T-shaped, 7.5-MHz, 8-cm intraoperative transducer (Aloka).

a sector transducer, but this reduces near-field visualization and may make appreciation of segmental anatomy more difficult, particularly for surgeons not used to looking at ultrasound images.

A 5.0 or 7.5 MHz frequency can be used. Penetration to the back of the liver may be impaired with a 7.5 MHz transducer, but this can be overcome by lifting the liver and scanning from underneath.

A console which can be sterilized may be an advantage to those operators who prefer to manipulate the controls themselves. However, not only is it time-consuming to sterilize both machine and probes, but this requires planning ahead, which is not always possible with some theatre lists. Scrupulous cleaning postoperatively is also essential. In comparison, by using a second (possibly unskilled) operator for the manipulation of the controls IOUS can be performed on demand at short notice and with great success using an unsterilized machine.

METHODS

It is absolutely essential that the operator is skilled in ultrasound techniques, to enable good technique and machine settings to be employed, to maximize the information received from the scan and to interpret the images correctly. Although some surgeons possess the necessary skills, there is an obvious role in IOUS for the sonographer.

In our institution, the sonographer scrubs in order to perform the scan. It is important to position the ultrasound monitor high enough to allow comfortable visualization from the operating field. Subdued light should be used, while still leaving enough light over the operating table. The ultrasound machine is first prepared by setting the controls, including time gain compensation (TGC), power, scale and orientation at an appropriate level. Manipulation of the few necessary controls after the sonographer has scrubbed can be easily performed, under instruction, by a non-sterile member of staff. The alternative to this method is for the sonographer to operate the controls while instructing the surgeon how to scan. This latter option is never quite as successful and can lead to severe sonographer and surgeon frustration.

The transducer is placed inside a sterile sheath containing coupling gel. The sheath should be long enough to cover a considerable length of the cable in order to avoid contamination of the sterile field.

The transducer can then be placed directly on the liver surface, as the natural moisture makes any coupling medium unnecessary. Note, however, that surface metastases do cause lack of contact. The liver is fully interrogated, both longitudinally from left to right and superior to inferior, and transversely. It must be borne in mind that the planes of scan are not the same as those used percutaneously, which of necessity tend to be slightly oblique, using subcostal and intercostal approaches.

The liver is then scanned via an inferior approach, which overcomes problems of penetration due to the high frequency and identifies nodules on the anterior surface that may be otherwise obscured by near-field artefact. A saline stand-off may be useful for near-field visualization in some cases.

The position of any lesion is noted in relationship to the vascular anatomy (Figures 16.2 and 16.3). The segmental anatomy is established by scanning the portal and hepatic veins.

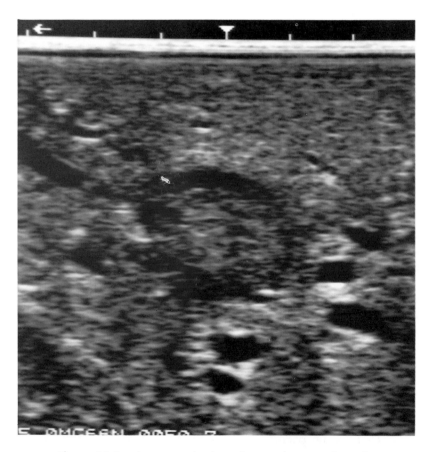

Figure 16.2   A metastatic deposit near the porta hepatis.

The average scanning time involved during a liver resection is approximately 5–10 minutes.

DISCUSSION

The many advantages of IOUS are associated with its superior resolution, dynamic nature and mobility of equipment. Intraoperative ultrasound has been consistently proven to identify small lesions in the liver which were undetected during conventional preoperative staging.

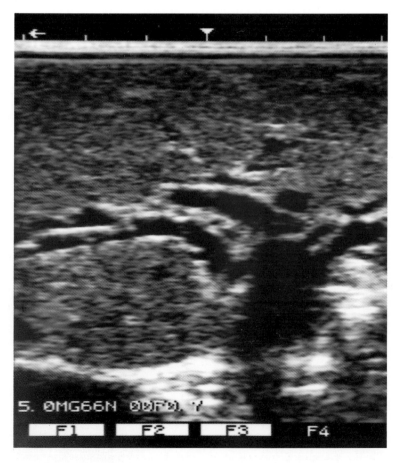

Figure 16.3 Same patient as Figure 16.2, showing dilated intrahepatic ducts at the porta from portal lymphadenopathy.

In addition to confirming preoperative findings at the time of surgery (which is particularly useful if there has been a delay between preoperative imaging and surgery), IOUS is able to accurately locate lesions in relation to vessels and segmental anatomy within the liver. The 'immediacy' of this dynamic technique is of great advantage to the surgeon, who is able to make prompt, well-informed decisions and change the surgical approach if necessary. The proposed line of resection can be examined and modified if appropriate, allowing clear margins to be left around the resected area. In some cases resection is abandoned as a result of multiple, previously undetected lesions found on IOUS.

IOUS differentiates solid lesions from small cysts when preoperative imaging is equivocal, and allows biopsy where necessary. Vasculature

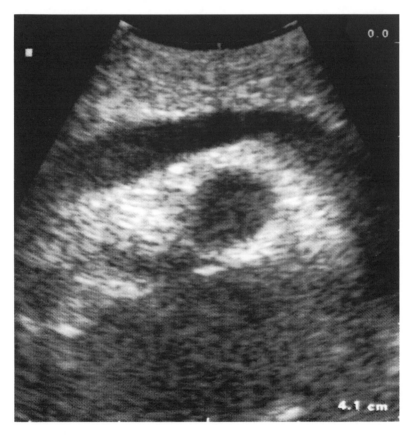

Figure 16.4   Laparoscopic image of the body of the pancreas.

within the liver may be inspected for infiltration and occlusion by adjacent tumour, as there is a worse prognosis with vascular invasion. In addition, other organs, such as pancreas (Figure 16.4) and kidneys, are readily accessible and extrahepatic tumour may be detected in some cases.

IOUS alone has been found significantly to affect the course of surgery in 42% of cases (Machi et al., 1987) with a consequent favourable alteration of the prognosis. In our series, around 70% of patients

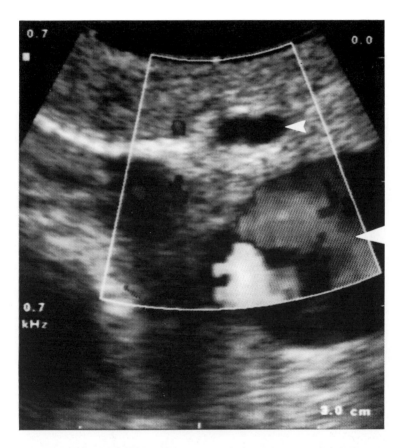

Figure 16.5 Laparoscopic ultrasound of the lower end of the normal calibre common bile duct (CBD) (small arrow) in a patient undergoing laparoscopic cholecystectomy for gallstones. Colour Doppler (seen in the portal vein; large arrow) was helpful in differentiating the CBD from adjacent blood vessels.

remain tumour-free 12 months after resection for metastases from various primary carcinomas.

It is necessary for the operator to be trained and skilled in the use of ultrasound, and it is therefore advantageous if the sonographer is able to scrub and perform the scan directly. Close co-operation between the surgical team and the sonographer is obviously necessary for this, but any initial reservations are soon dispelled. The superior quality, and speed, of the ultrasound examination by a skilled operator has obvious advantages, and if the sonographer can be warned in advance of the procedure no additional operating time is used in preparation.

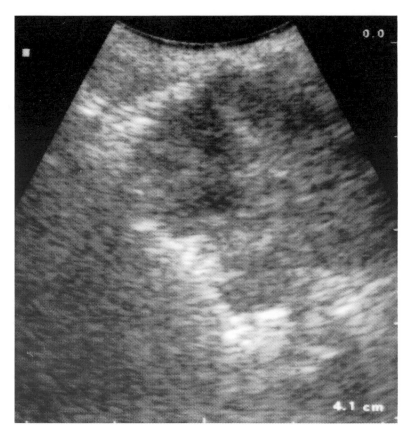

Figure 16.6   A laparoscopic ultrasound image of a 2.8 cm colonic primary carcinoma medial to the right lobe of the liver. This lesion was highly vascular on colour flow Doppler.

No other imaging modality offers such advantages in this situation and, therefore, the role of IOUS looks set to expand, particularly with the gradually (if cautiously) increasing popularity of hepatic resection. IOUS in this field directly affects the success of the treatment and offers a change in the prognosis for many patients.

Future trends may include the use of colour Doppler (Figure 16.5) and hepatic contrast media. Little is known about the effects of these techniques in IOUS, and it is difficult at this stage to predict how, if at all, they could improve upon the already dramatic impact of high-resolution IOUS. Laparoscopic ultrasound is also gaining acceptance in staging (Figures 16.6 and 16.7), and potentially reduces morbidity

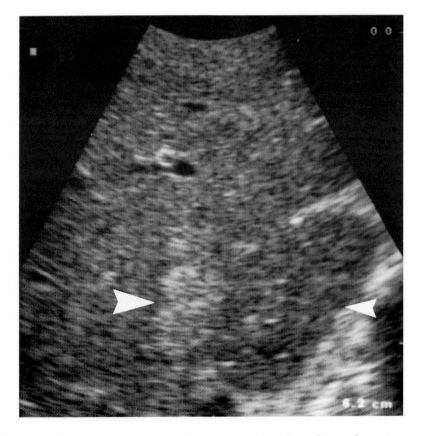

Figure 16.7   Metastatic deposit (large arrow) from the colorectal carcinoma shown in Figure 16.4 in the right lobe of the liver adjacent to the right kidney (small arrow). This was not demonstrable on preoperative imaging.

from large incisions in patients who turn out to be inoperable. Recently, cryotherapy has been introduced into the surgical procedure for smaller tumours, although its usefulness has yet to be proven. Increasing attention is also being paid to the use of laser therapy and percutaneous alcohol ablation of metastases (Amin et al., 1993).

The sonographer's role in IOUS is likely to become the accepted trend, and sonographer involvement in these techniques will certainly ensure the continuing development of IOUS in the detection of focal nodules, in determining their relationship to vasculature and in guidance for diagnostic and therapeutic techniques.

References

Adson, M.A., Van Heerden, J.A., Adson, M.H. et al. (1984) Resection of hepatic metastases from colorectal cancer. *Archives of Surgery* **119:** 647–651.

Amin, Z., Bown, S.G., Lees, W.R. (1993) Local treatment of colorectal liver metastases: a comparison of interstitial laser photocoagulation (ILP) and percutaneous alcohol injection (PAI). *Clinical Radiology* **48:** 166–171.

Bengmark, S., Hafstrom, L. (1978) The natural course of liver cancer. *Progress in Clinical Cancer* **7:** 195.

Freeny, P.C., Marks, W.M. (1986) Patterns of contrast enhancement of benign and malignant hepatic neoplasms during bolus dynamic and delayed CT. *Radiology* **160:** 613–618.

Heiken, J.P., Weyman, P.J., Lee, J.K.T. (1989) Detection of focal hepatic masses: prospective evaluation with CT, delayed CT, CT during arterial portography, and MR imaging. *Radiology* **171:** 47–51.

Kane, R.A., Hughes, L.A., Cua, E.J. et al. (1994) The impact of intraoperative ultrasonography on surgery for liver neoplasms. *Journal of Ultrasound Medicine* **13:** 1–6.

Knol, J.A., Marn, C.S., Francis, I.R. et al. (1993) Comparisons of dynamic infusion and delayed computed tomography, intraoperative ultrasound, and palpation in the diagnosis of liver metastases. *American Journal of Surgery* **165:** 81–87.

Machi, J., Isomoto, H., Yamashita, Y. et al. (1987) Intraoperative ultrasonography in screening for liver metastases from colorectal cancer: comparative accuracy with traditional procedures. *Surgery* **101:** 678–684.

Machi, J., Isomoto, H., Kurohiji, T. et al. (1991) Accuracy of intraoperative ultrasonography in diagnosing liver metastasis from colorectal cancer: evaluation with postoperative follow-up results. *World Journal of Surgery* **15:** 551–557.

Russo, A., Sparacino, G. (1989) Role of intraoperative ultrasound in the screening of liver metastases from colorectal carcinoma: initial experiences. *Journal of Surgical Oncology* **42:** 249–255.

Semelka, R.C., Shoenut, J.P., Kroeker, M.A. et al. (1992) Focal liver disease: comparison of dynamic contrast-enhanced CT and T2 weighted fat-suppressed FLASH, and gadolinium-enhanced MR imaging at 1.5 T1. *Radiology* **184:** 687–694.

Stewart, P., Chu, J.M., Kos, S.C. et al. (1993) Intra-operative ultrasound for the detection of hepatic metastases from colorectal cancer. *Australian and New Zealand Journal of Surgery* **63:** 530–534.

Sugarbaker, P.H., Kemeny, N. (1988) Management of metastatic liver cancer. *Advances in Surgery* **22:** 1–55.

17

Magnetic Resonance Imaging Investigation of Arachnoiditis

Elizabeth M. Warren

INTRODUCTION

Arachnoiditis is a challenging and controversial field both for the clinical diagnostician and the imaging department. Clinical diagnosis is fraught with difficulty, since there is no characteristic symptom complex. In many patients there are multiple causative factors and a specific aetiology cannot be established.

Recent advances in magnetic resonance imaging (MRI) technology have produced marked improvements in image quality whilst reducing examination time. Thus with careful attention to technique, it is now feasible to non-invasively image the individual nerve roots of the cauda equina with sufficient resolution to detect arachnoiditis.

In this chapter, after reviewing the pathology and imaging appearances of arachnoiditis, the practical details and pitfalls of the MRI technique are described. Finally, the medico-legal implications of the diagnosis will be discussed.

WHAT IS ARACHNOIDITIS?

The mechanism of adhesive arachnoiditis is similar to the repair response of injury to serous membranes such as peritoneum, pericardium and pleura (Smolik and Nash, 1951; Quiles et al., 1978).

Unlike other inflammatory responses, arachnoiditis is initially characterized by a fibrinous exudate with a very minimal vascular inflammatory cellular reaction (Johnson and Sze, 1990). Very few enzyme-bearing leucocytes are released from the cells, due to the absence of hypervascularization. The phagocytes and fibrolytic enzymes that are present are probably diluted by the cerebrospinal fluid (CSF) and washed away, leaving the arachnoid incapable of eradicating these fibrinous bands. Consequently, the fibrin-covered nerve roots and arachnoid membrane (thecal sac) adhere to one another. These bands act as bridges and supports for the proliferating fibrocytes to lay down collagen during the stage of repair. This results in the formation of collagenized adhesions (Quiles et al., 1978). Thus the term 'adhesive arachnoiditis' applies to the end-stage of repair of arachnoid inflammation.

CAUSES

Chronic adhesive arachnoiditis has a variety of causes, including agents injected into the subarachnoid space such as contrast media, anaesthetics and intradural steroids. Infection, trauma, surgery and intrathecal haemorrhage are also all potential causes of the condition (Quiles et al., 1978). The use of the intrathecal oil-based contrast agents such as iodophendylate (Myodil or Pantopaque) has been implicated as a major cause (Occleshaw, 1987). This positive myelographic contrast medium was used from the mid-1940s until non-ionic water-soluble media took its place during the early 1980s.

SYMPTOMS

The clinical diagnosis of arachnoiditis is difficult because it has no distinct symptom complex (Jorgensen et al., 1975; Burton, 1978; Quiles et al., 1978). The condition is most commonly found in patients with chronic unremitting back pain and radiating leg pain following either surgery and/or myelography for lumbar disc disease.

NORMAL APPEARANCES OF LUMBAR NERVE ROOTS

Adhesive arachnoiditis affects the distribution and appearance of the nerve roots, which is best seen on axial imaging of the spine. The distribution of normal roots of the cauda equina shows considerable variation between subjects. Consequently accurate interpretation of abnormal studies requires an understanding of the normal range of appearance at each vertebral level (Ross et al., 1987; Cohen et al., 1991).

The images and corresponding diagrams shown in Figures 17.1–17.5 represent a likely distribution in a 'normal' subject.

THE IMAGING APPEARANCE OF ARACHNOIDITIS

Myelography and Postmyelogram CT

The appearance of arachnoiditis is well known on both myelography and postmyelogram computed tomography (CT), representing the 'gold standard' in its diagnosis (Jorgensen et al., 1975; Delamarter et al., 1990; Johnson and Sze, 1990). Arachnoiditis is a progressive process (Burton, 1978) and therefore shows a variety of appearances on imaging, including a homogeneous contrast pattern without root shadows and subarachnoid filling defects with narrowing and shortening of the thecal sac. Two groups of patients have been described based on the severity of the myelographic findings (Jorgensen et al., 1975):

1. *Type 1*, or mild disease, cases show thickened 'sleeveless' nerve roots caused by adhesions of the roots to the inside of the meninges (Figure 17.6).
2. *Type 2*, or more extensive disease, cases present with myelographic filling defects, narrowing, shortening and occlusion of the thecal sac. As the clumping becomes more prominent and the thecal sac and roots become one soft-tissue mass a complete myelographic block can result. This is considered as the 'end-stage' of adhesive arachnoiditis (Figure 17.7).

On postmyelogram CT the clumping of the nerve roots can be directly visualized. The adherence of the nerve roots to the thecal sac produces a featureless or 'empty sac' appearance.

Magnetic Resonance Imaging

The findings of arachnoiditis have also been described and classified using MRI (Ross et al., 1987) and there is good correlation with the myelographic and postmyelogram CT appearances (Ross et al., 1987;

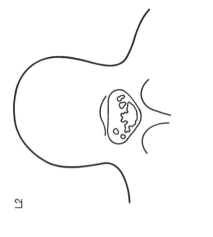

L2

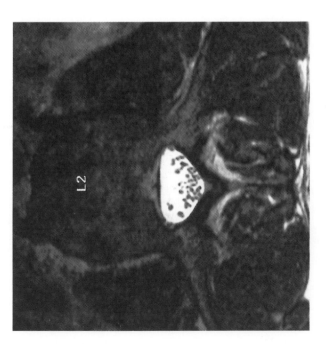

L2

Figure 17.1 The roots occupy most of the thecal sac at the level of L2, assuming a smooth crescentric appearance after the curvature of the sac.

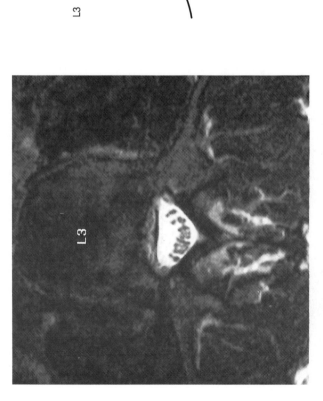

L3

L3

Figure 17.2 The roots at L3 are grouped and amassed posteriorly, being either crescentric or, sometimes, irregular in appearance. The exiting roots can usually be seen anterolaterally in a symmetric configuration.

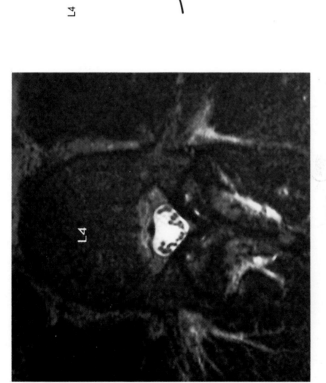

L4

Figure 17.3 The roots at L4 are often sufficiently dispersed that they are seen as separate entities arranged in a symmetric pattern within the CSF.

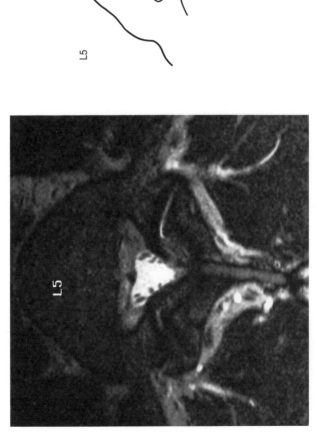

Figure 17.4 At L5 fewer roots are evident and tend to be equally spaced from one another within the thecal sac. A pattern of conglomeration at the centre of the sac seen at the other levels is lacking at this lower level.

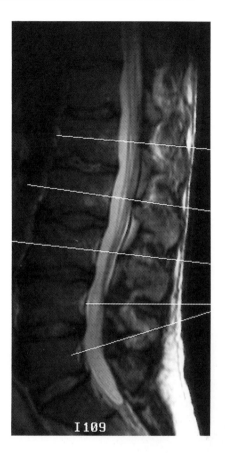

Figure 17.5   Sagittal T2 weighted image showing the position of the axial slices pictured in Figures 17.1–17.4, demonstrating the normal appearances of the lumbar nerve roots.

Delamarter et al., 1990). The MRI findings may be classified into three categories or patterns (Ross, 1991):

1. *Group 1* shows central adhesion of the nerve roots within the thecal sac seen as a central clump of soft-tissue signal. Instead of demonstrating a normal feathery pattern the nerve roots are clumped into one or more cords (Figure 17.8).
2. *Group 2* shows adhesion of the nerve roots to the meninges giving rise to an 'empty sac' sign. The MRI depicts only the homogeneous

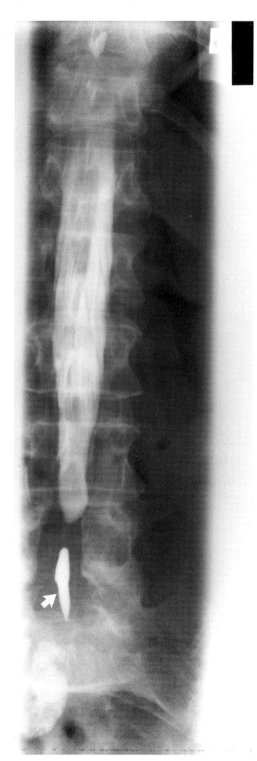

Figure 17.6 The myelographic appearance of arachnoiditis demonstrating the thickened 'sleeveless' nerve roots associated with type-1 disease. A small amount of residual Myodil can also be seen on this image (arrow).

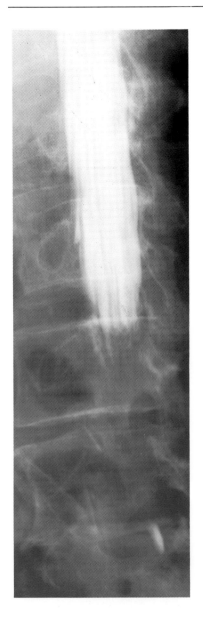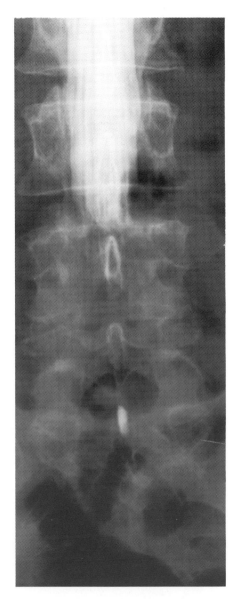

Figure 17.7 The myelographic appearance of a more severe type-2 case, demonstrating a complete block of contrast caused by the amassed nerve roots.

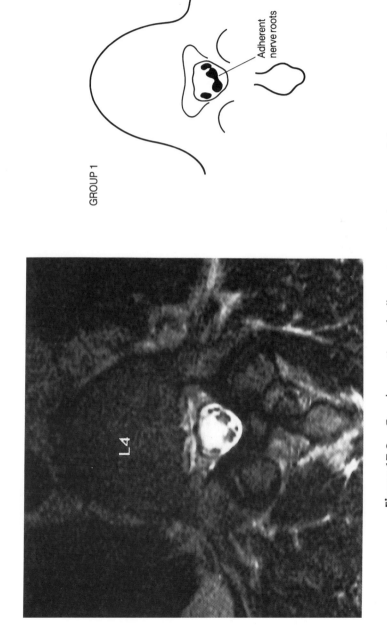

Figure 17.8 Conglomeration of adherent roots in the centre of the sac.

signal from the CSF within the thecal sac, whilst the nerve roots are peripherally attached to the meninges (Figure 17.9).

3. *Group 3* constitutes the 'end-stage' of the inflammatory response; here the arachnoiditis becomes an inflammatory mass that fills the thecal sac, appearing as a non-specific soft-tissue mass (Figure 17.10).

It is important to note that in the individual patient there can be a spectrum of appearances evident due to the progressive nature of the disease with one or more patterns being demonstrated. For example, central and peripheral clumping often occur together (Ross, 1991).

Contrast Enhanced MRI

In most cases there is little enhancement of arachnoiditis with the use of intravenous contrast such as gadolinium diethylene triaminepenta-acetic acid (DTPA) (Ross, 1991). It has been suggested that subtle enhancement may be more easily appreciated with the use of fat suppression (Tien et al., 1992). However, there is usually much less enhancement in arachnoiditis, even at the 'inflammatory mass' stage, than would occur with a neoplasm.

THE APPEARANCE OF RESIDUAL MYODIL/PANTOPAQUE ON MRI

Focal collections of Myodil or Pantopaque in the thecal sac have a characteristic appearance on MRI. They display high signal intensity on T1 weighted images and low signal intensity on T2 weighted images (Braun et al., 1986; Mamourian and Briggs, 1986) (Figure 17.11).

It is possible to confuse residual Myodil with lipoma due to their similar appearance (Braun et al., 1986), but the two can usually be distinguished by the use of a short tau inversion recovery (STIR) sequence which nulls the fat signal intensity of the lipoma but not the Myodil due to their different T1 relaxation times.

DIFFICULTIES IN IDENTIFYING ARACHNOIDITIS ON MRI

There are difficulties in identifying arachnoiditis using MRI (Ross, 1991). These are as follows:

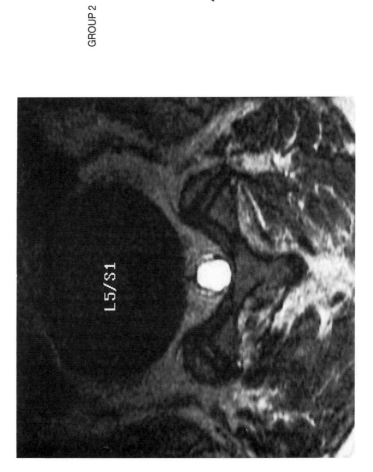

GROUP 2

Adherent nerve roots

L5/S1

Figure 17.9 Thickened nerve roots adherent to the periphery of the thecal sac – 'empty sac' appearance.

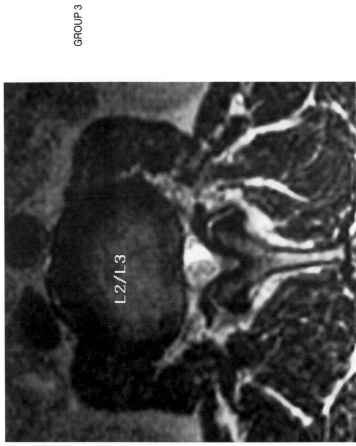

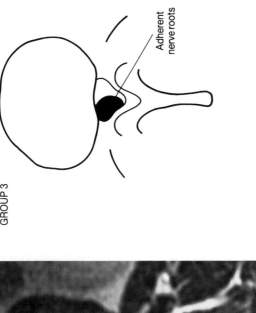

GROUP 3

Adherent
nerve roots

Figure 17.10 A soft-tissue mass partially obliterating the subarachnoid space.

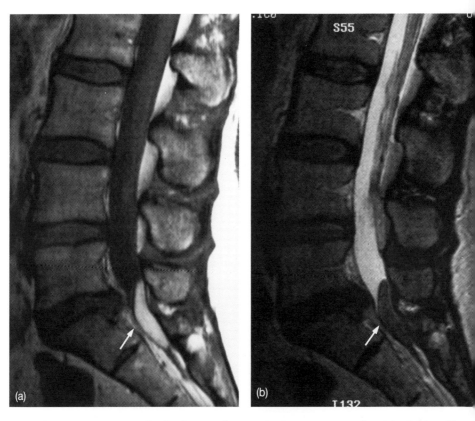

Figure 17.11 (a) The high signal intensity appearance of residual Myodil on a sagittal T1 weighted image. (b) The same patient with the low signal intensity appearance of Myodil on a T2 weighted image.

1. In differentiating an inflammatory mass from an intradural neoplasm as the two can look identical on magnetic resonance (MR) images (Vloeberghs et al, 1992). The patient's history obviously needs to be taken into account in determining the diagnosis, along with the fact that enhancement with gadolinium is less intense in arachnoiditis than in a neoplasm.
2. CSF tumour spread and the central clumping pattern of arachnoiditis can appear similar. Arachnoiditis tends to be smooth and fairly symmetrical in appearance, whereas drop metastases are more irregular in pattern and also enhance to a greater degree than arachnoiditis.
3. Bony canal stenosis may give a similar pattern to central clumping

due to arachnoiditis. However, usually the extradural degenerative disease that is causing the compression is easily demonstrated on MRI.
4. Although the diagnosis of moderate to severe cases of arachnoiditis is well proven on MRI, mild cases are much more difficult. In these cases myelography is still the most sensitive technique and remains the 'gold standard'.

MR TECHNIQUE IN THE INVESTIGATION OF ARACHNOIDITIS

Prior to the advent of MRI, the diagnosis of arachnoiditis was made by myelography and postmyelogram CT. In the late 1980s, surface-coil MRI with slice thicknesses of less than 5 mm was found to be capable of defining individual nerve roots within the thecal sac (Ross et al., 1987). The presentation on MRI was shown to be of a very similar pattern to that seen on CT myelography. A number of studies have demonstrated excellent correlation of moderate to severe cases between MRI and both myelography and CT myelography (Ross et al., 1987; Delamarter et al., 1990; Johnson and Sze, 1990). It was also suggested that MRI could replace invasive investigations (Johnson and Sze, 1990).

MRI technology has progressed rapidly since this time resulting in a dramatic improvement in image resolution and reduced scan times. The progressive nature of the disease and spectrum of appearances encountered, further compounded by the variable distribution of nerve roots in the 'normal' subject, mean that a high-quality imaging technique is required. The pulse sequence and imaging parameters need to be selected to maximize image quality, with the emphasis on high resolution whilst still maintaining a good signal-to-noise ratio (Modic et al., 1994). The resolution that is required to reliably diagnose nerve root clumping is only practically achieved with the use of 512 matrix, as the accompanying examples demonstrate (see Figure 17.15). These conditions are most easily achieved with the use of a high-field system.

The most important images necessary to make the diagnosis are those undertaken in the axial plane. However, in order to localize accurately and diagnose any other pathology that may be the cause of the symptoms, it is necessary to include two sagittal sequences, one T1 and the other T2 weighted (Figure 17.12). These should also be of a good image quality, making use of high resolution wherever possible within the constraints of a reasonable examination time. An example of the

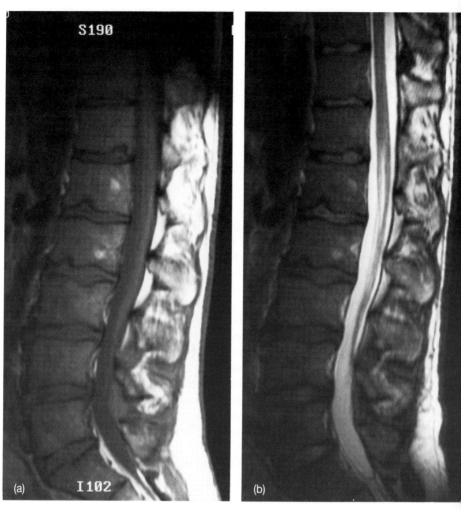

S190

I102

(a)   (b)

Figure 17.12   (a) An example of a T1 weighted 'fast spin echo' midline sagittal image performed as part of the protocol used for investigating arachnoiditis. (b) The midline sagittal image of the T2 weighted 'fast spin echo' sequence. The imaging parameters used for these sequences are given in Table 17.1.

imaging parameters used for each sequence undertaken on a 1.5-T GE Signa is included in Table 17.1 for reference.

The literature provides some debate on the choice of sequence weighting for the axial images. Axial T1 weighted images are preferred

Table 17.1   1.5-T MRI system (GE Signa)

Parameter	Sagittal T1W	Sagittal T2W	Axial/oblique T2W
Sequence	Fast spin echo	Fast spin echo	Fast spin echo
Echo time (ms)	16	96	100
Repetition time (ms)	600	3460	6280
Matrix	512 × 256	512 × 256	512 × 256
Number of excitations/ signal averages	2	2	2
Field of view (cm)	38	38	22
Slice thickness/skip (mm)	4/1	4/1	4
Options	Presaturation, superior/ inferior	Presaturation, superior/ inferior	Presaturation, superior/inferior, right/left; No phase wrap
Echo-train length	4	16	16
Time (min:s)	2:36	1:58	3:21

by some, particularly in demonstrating pathology in type-3 patients, whilst others find that greater contrast is provided on T2 weighted axial scans in defining the distribution of the individual nerve roots (Ross et al., 1987). Recent practice has found that T2 weighted axial images are the most effective in diagnosing arachnoiditis, particularly with the use of the faster spin echo pulse sequences now available. Figure 17.13 demonstrates an example from a group of axial/oblique images undertaken with a 512 × 384 matrix, achieving 15 slices in a scan time of 5 minutes. In addition to high-resolution T2 weighted axial images, a diagnosis necessitates visualizing the appearance of the roots over several levels, ideally encompassing a range from the level of D11 to S1 (Modic et al., 1994). Figure 17.14 shows an example of slice prescription suitable to achieve the necessary coverage.

The importance of high-resolution MRI cannot be overemphasized, as the following examples will demonstrate. A 'normal' subject was scanned on two MRI systems of different field strengths and a comparison was made between the clarity of the axial T2 weighted images produced. The parameters used for the images produced at 0.5 T are shown in Table 17.2, correlating reasonably well with those used at 1.5 T. Using the high-field-strength system only, axial T2 weighted scans were undertaken utilizing a range of image matrices, maintaining all other imaging parameters constant, as shown in Table 17.1. The images produced to demonstrate this comparison are shown in Figure 17.15 along with a localizer showing the slice position of the image that was selected.

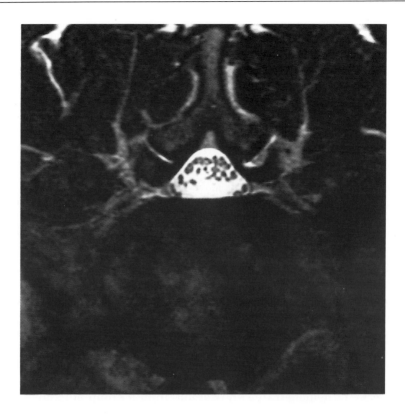

Figure 17.13   An example of an axial/oblique T2 weighted image at L2/3, demonstrating a high level of image quality achieved with the use of 512 matrix on a 1.5-T MRI system.

Table 17.2   0.5-T MRI system

Parameter	Axial/oblique T2
Sequence	Turbo spin echo
Echo time (ms)	150
Repetition time (ms)	3574
Matrix	512 × 245
Number of excitations/ signal averages	8
Field of view (cm)	35
Slice thickness (mm)	4
Options	No phase wrap
Turbo factor	19
Scan time (min:s)	5:22

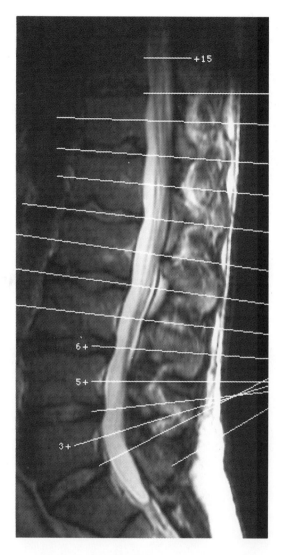

Figure 17.14 A sagittal T2 weighted 'fast spin echo' midline image, demonstrating the position and orientation of the axial/oblique slices. It is important to note that coverage is achieved from D11 to S1.

It is clear from comparing the images that, even with the use of modern MRI systems with advanced coil technology, a wide range of image quality and resolving power may be produced. It is therefore vitally important when undertaking an examination to detect adhesive

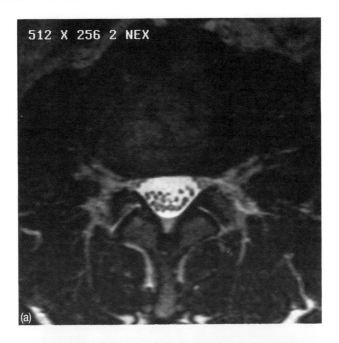

512 X 256 2 NEX

(a)

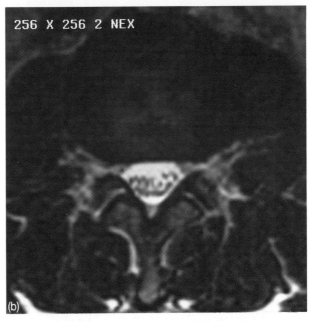

256 X 256 2 NEX

(b)

Figure 17.15   (caption overleaf)

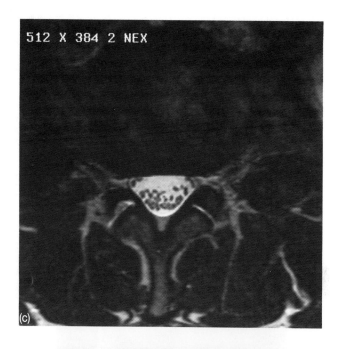

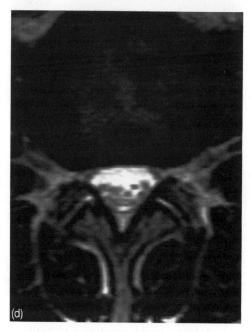

Figure 17.15 (caption overleaf)

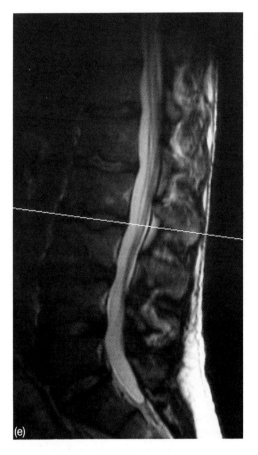

Figure 17.15   (a) T2 weighted, fast spin echo, 1.5-T GE Signa, quadrature spine coil, 512 × 256 matrix, 2 nex. This image represents the minimum resolution that is required for reliable visualization of the individual nerve roots. (b) T2 weighted, fast spin echo, 1.5-T GE Signa, quadrature spine coil, 256 × 256 matrix, 2 nex. It is much more difficult to identify the individual nerve roots on this image compared to (a) and (c). (c) T2 weighted, fast spin echo, 1.5-T GE Signa, quadrature spine coil, 512 × 384 matrix, 2 nex. This image demonstrates the improvement in resolution that can be obtained with a finer matrix and an increase in scan time of under 2 minutes. (d) T2 weighted, fast spin echo, 0.5-T MRI system, quadrature spine coil, 512 × 245 matrix, 8 nex. The individual nerve roots are not seen as reliably at 0.5 T as they are at 1.5 T, despite the use of a high-resolution matrix. (e) Sagittal, T2 weighted image showing the position of the slice selected for comparison of the different techniques.

arachnoiditis that these points of technique are given priority. Figure 17.15(a) demonstrates the minimum image quality and resolution required for the reliable differentiation of individual nerve roots.

THE CURRENT INVESTIGATION OF ARACHNOIDITIS

Recent interest has focused on the extent to which Myodil used in lumbar myelography could be responsible for chronic adhesive arachnoiditis. The answer to this is as yet unknown as the clinical picture is so often complicated by the back disease itself and, therefore, other possible causes.

However, experimental studies on animals have shown that injection of drugs including contrast media into the subarachnoid space can cause acute and chronic inflammation of the meninges (Howland and Curry, 1966). The combination of blood and contrast medium has also been implicated in increasing the incidence of arachnoiditis as has myelography followed by surgery (Occleshaw, 1987).

In an attempt to resolve this issue, a number of retrospective studies have been undertaken on patients who have had Myodil introduced by ventriculography or cisternography remote from the lumbar spine (Hughes and Isherwood, 1992; Rowland Hill et al., 1992). These studies could not identify any definite correlation that Myodil alone was responsible for causing symptomatic chronic arachnoiditis.

Despite the continued uncertainty regarding the exact role of Myodil in causation of symptomatic arachnoiditis, there has been very little recent research on this subject. Currently, a number of patients in the UK who were subjected to Myodil myelography are pursuing a claim for compensation against the manufacturer of the contrast agent. This group, as part of the action, are undergoing a rigorous clinical examination. In addition many patients are receiving assessment by MRI in order to establish whether they meet the criteria for a diagnosis of symptomatic post-Myodil arachnoiditis.

The role of MRI in this study is to document accurately the extent and severity of the disease and exclude extradural causes. It has been postulated that arachnoiditis found at a level remote from any surgery and the lumbosacral junction is more likely to be significant. The successful assessment of the MR images is dependent on a comprehensive study using a high-resolution technique, as described previously. The investigation of these patients is at present reaching completion. The results and conclusions drawn from this study should prove very valuable in the assessment of the symptomatic disease and its link with oil-based contrast media.

Myodil has already been the subject of medical litigation when in 1971 an Appeal ruling in the USA adjudged a physician negligent for non-removal of the contrast (Occleshaw, 1987). It remains to be decided whether the claim against the manufacturer of Myodil will be successful and the contrast agent implicated legally as a cause for symptomatic adhesive arachnoiditis.

Acknowledgements

The author thanks Lyn Hamilton for her secretarial assistance and Dr A. J. Molyneux for advice and myelography images. General thanks to Dr M. J. Warren, Mary Dingley and the staff at the Oxford MRI Centre, John Radcliffe Hospital.

References

Braun, I.F., Malko, J.A., Davis, P.C. et al. (1986) The behaviour of Pantopaque on MR: in vivo and in vitro analyses. *American Journal of Neuroradiology* **7:** 997–1001.

Burton, C.V. (1978) Lumbosacral arachnoiditis. *Spine* **3:** 24–30.

Cohen, M.S., Wall, E.J., Kerber, C.W. et al. (1991) The anatomy of the cauda equina on CT scans and MRI. *Journal of Bone and Joint Surgery* **73B:** 381–384.

Delamarter, R.B., Ross, J.S., Marsaryk, T.J. et al. (1990) Diagnosis of lumbar arachnoiditis by magnetic resonance imaging. *Spine* **15:** 304–310.

Howland, W.J., Curry, J.L. (1966) Experimental studies of Pantopaque arachnoiditis. *Radiology* **87:** 253–261.

Hughes, D.G., Isherwood, I. (1992) How frequent is chronic lumbar arachnoiditis following intrathecal Myodil? *British Journal of Radiology* **65:** 758–760.

Johnson, C.E., Sze, G. (1990) Benign lumbar arachnoiditis: MR imaging with Gadopentetate Dimeglumine. *American Journal of Neuroradiology* **11:** 763–770.

Jorgensen, J., Hansen, P.H., Steenskov, V., Oveson, N. (1975) A clinical and radiological study of chronic lower spinal arachnoiditis. *Neuroradiology* **9:** 139–144.

Mamourian, A.C., Briggs, R.W. (1986) Appearances of Pantopaque on MR images. *Radiology* **158:** 457–460.

Occleshaw, J.V. (1987) Myelography and cisternography. In Ansell, G., Wilkins, R.A. (eds) *Complications in Diagnostic Imaging*, 2nd edn, pp 313–314. Oxford: Blackwell.

Quiles, M., Marchisello, P.J., Tsairis, P. (1978) Lumbar adhesive arachnoiditis. *Spine* **3:** 45–50.

Ross, J.S. (1991) Magnetic resonance assessment of the postoperative spine. *Radiologic Clinics of North America* **29:** 793–808.

Ross, J.S., Marsaryk, T.J., Modic, M.T. et al. (1987) MR imaging of lumbar arachnoiditis. *American Journal of Roentgenology* **149:** 1025–1032.

Ross, J.S. (1994) Inflammatory disease. In: Modic, M.T., Marsaryk, T.J., Ross, J.S. (eds) *MRI of the Spine*, 2nd edn, pp 216–223. St Louis, Missouri: Mosby.

Rowland Hill, C.A., Hunter, J.V., Moseley, I.F. et al. (1992) Does Myodil introduced for ventriculography lead to symptomatic lumbar arachnoiditis? *British Journal of Radiology* **65:** 1105–1107.

Smolik, E., Nash, F. (1951) Lumbar spinal arachnoiditis: a complication of the intervertebral disc operation. *Annals of Surgery* **133:** 490–495.

Tien, R.D., Olson, E.M., Zee, C.S. (1992) Diseases of the lumbar spine: findings on fat-suppression MR imaging. *American Journal of Roentgenology* **159:** 95–99.

Vloeberghs, M., Herregodts, P., Stadnik, T. et al. (1992) Spinal arachnoiditis mimicking a spinal cord tumour: a case report and review of the literature. *Surgery and Neurology* **37:** 211–215.

18

Pseudo-dynamic Magnetic Resonance Imaging in Orthopaedics

Susan G. Moore

INTRODUCTION

Joint pain is often described by a patient as positional, or elicited only during a specific movement or activity. Imaging of any kind, in a neutral position, is therefore unlikely to elucidate the problem. Magnetic resonance imaging (MRI) is an excellent technique for looking at soft-tissue structures and their morphological changes on movement, and hence pseudo-dynamic or 'kinematic' MRI can be a powerful tool in visualizing functional anatomy. Reviewing current literature reveals that the use of MRI for pseudo-dynamics is increasing, but techniques are constantly being refined and applied into new areas.

All pseudo-dynamic imaging requires non-ferromagnetic positioning apparatus that will allow the required joint movement, whilst restricting involuntary motion. At the same time, the range of joint movement must not be inhibited by the positioning apparatus or by application of any outside force or mass (hence the term 'kinematic').

Scanning sequences used must spatially resolve the relevant anatomy, whilst maintaining a realistic examination time for the patient. For this reason, short echo spin echoes (T1 weighted) and fast spin echo or fast gradient echo sequences are optimal at present.

True dynamic studies are becoming possible with current sequences but with limited application, so those described in this chapter are the best approximation so far of joint motion. Static images are scanned incrementally through the range of motion of a joint and then visualized in a 'cine-loop' formation which is a function of most scanner software. This allows evaluation of normal and abnormal alignment of joints in relation to their movement and any underlying or secondary pathology.

At present, pseudo-dynamic techniques are most frequently applied to the temporomandibular joint and the patellofemoral joint. There has been some success with the wrist, cervical spine, shoulder and ankle. This chapter reviews the techniques and development of pseudo-dynamic MRI and its applications.

THE WRIST

Applications:
1. Carpal motion.
2. Instability patterns.
3. Impingement.
4. Movement abnormalities.

High-resolution images of the wrist demand a small surface coil, most usually a circular 'receive only' coil in single or dual configuration. Reported pseudo-dynamic studies have described T1-weighted spin echo imaging in the axial or coronal planes (Olerud et al., 1988; Shellock et al., 1991a). When scanning in the coronal plane the patient is positioned prone, with the arm extended above the shoulder. Padding is used for comfort and immobilization and the wrist can be positioned in a special apparatus that both aids immobilization and allows the wrist to move in increments from radial to neutral to ulnar deviated positions (Figure 18.1).

Earlier studies had used axial plane imaging, the forearm moving from pronation to neutral to supination positions (Olerud et al., 1988). The resulting information showed congruent movement of the radius around the ulnar head, previously only postulated by investigation in cadaver specimens.

Yoshioka et al. (1993) extended the previous work of Skie et al. (1990) using pseudo-dynamics to look at the morphology of the carpal tunnel shape. Any reduction in the area of the carpal tunnel can result in median nerve compression, increasing the pressure in the carpal tunnel. A significant increase in pressure is noted when the wrist is in

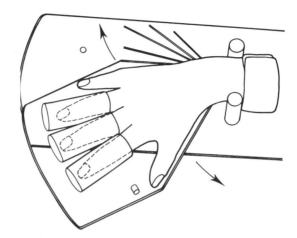

Figure 18.1   Example of a wrist-positioning device for pseudo-dynamic scanning.

extension. The technique described uses T1-weighted spin echo images in the axial plane. The wrist is scanned in neutral and splinted 40° flexion or splinted 50° extension. The cross-sectional area of the carpal tunnel is measured using computer analysis. Their results detail the changing shape of the carpal tunnel during wrist extension and flexion and they conclude that changes in morphology on wrist movement can increase intracarpal pressure, as well as factors such as canal stenosis or mass effect from space-occupying lesions (which are a direct result of median nerve compression). Therefore dynamic changes are a contributory factor to median nerve entrapment and carpal tunnel syndrome. Pseudo-dynamic MRI is the imaging tool of choice to view those dynamic changes in the wrist.

CERVICAL SPINE

Applications:
1. Lesions at craniocervical junction.
2. Anterior atlantoaxial subluxation.
3. Compression of upper cervical cord.
4. Rheumatoid arthritis (RA).

Pseudo-dynamic MRI of the cervical spine is limited at present, and reports compare the technique with plain lateral cervical spine X-rays. The technique described is usually a T1-weighted spin echo sequence in the sagittal plane, at the craniocervical junction. The cervical spine is scanned in neutral, flexion and extension positions. McAfee et al. (1986) suggested that pseudo-dynamic MRI of the cervical spine was the optimal examination where instability was present, as it showed the mechanism of compression. However, Kawaida et al. (1989) challenged that opinion. Their results of a pseudo-dynamic study showed that indentation of the neural tissues seen on the neutral image showed no significant changes on the extension image, where the degree of subluxation (anterior atlantoaxial) was reduced. They suggested that, where compression was demonstrated in the neutral position, pseudo-dynamic MRI in flexion and extension was unnecessary. They also concluded that compression of the medulla and upper cervical cord can quite adequately be evaluated from routine radiographs. These conclusions and the general lack of pseudo-dynamic MRI evaluation of the cervical spine suggest that the functional technique has had little impact in this area, to date.

THE SHOULDER

Applications:
1. Rotational abnormalities.
2. Tendon compression.
3. Labral motion.
4. Rotator cuff motion.

Pain in the shoulder joint is often positional, or apparent only on certain movement. Bonutti et al. (1993) have described a new positioning device which they devised, patent pending, to stabilize the humerus and allow increments of humeral rotation. The humerus is strapped into a brace which is connected to an 'indexer' that allows rotational movement in 10° increments. The indexer is patient-driven but can be overriden by the MRI operator. It is anchored to the couch so there is no shift during shoulder rotation and the shoulder and surface coil maintain their relative positions.

T2-weighted gradient echo images are scanned in the axial plane through the glenohumeral joint, in each position of rotation, using the full extent of internal to external rotation that the patient can manage. The resulting images are viewed in a cine-loop format, where the degrees of rotation can be measured as long as the bicipital groove is seen on each image. The technique enables visualization of rotation and translation of the humeral head in the glenoid, motion of the glenoid labrum and of the joint capsule. So far, the technique can identify normal positioning of the tendons and subsequent changes in position in patients with shoulder instability, as well as tendon compression and rotational abnormalities. The future of pseudo-dynamic MRI of the shoulder is promising; Bonutti et al. (1993) suggest that by using sequence modifications to permit more accurate anatomical definition of certain structures, labral motion and rotator cuff motion might be analysed.

THE ANKLE

Applications:
1. Bony structure.
2. Soft-tissue impingements.

Pseudo-dynamic MRI of the ankle joint is a relatively new technique and developmental work is ongoing. As with other small joints, high resolution is required to visualize small anatomical structures. For this reason Shellock et al. (1991a) recommend a dual 5-inch receive-only surface coil. They describe a technique with the patient supine and the ankle immobilized in a positioning device which allows ankle movement incrementally from dorsiflexion to neutral to plantar flexion. The mechanism is patient-activated. T1-weighted spin echo images are scanned in the sagittal plane at each position increment, with the resulting images viewed statically or in a cine-loop format.

Visualizing bony anatomy and ligaments that stabilize the joint, abnormalities of either can be seen on the static magnetic resonance (MR) image and any resultant misalignment of the ankle joint surfaces, on the pseudo-dynamic study. Joint surface displacements can produce secondary pathology in the joint. Pseudo-dynamic MRI of the ankle is excellent for soft-tissue impingement syndromes that affect plantar or dorsiflexion of the joint, while pathology such as osteochondritis dissecans and loose bodies and their effect on the dynamic function of the joint are well seen. Overall, evaluation of pseudo-dynamic MRI in the ankle joint is in its very early stages.

THE TEMPOROMANDIBULAR JOINT

Applications:
1. Internal derangement.

2. Asymmetrical motion.
3. Meniscal disc displacement and movement.

Anterior displacement of the meniscal disc in relation to the mandibular condyle is the most common internal derangement of the temporomandibular joint (TMJ) and pseudo-dynamic MRI is an excellent technique for demonstrating these displacements. Positioning devices are used that open the patient's mouth incrementally (patient-activated), with MR images taken at each of the mouth positions (Figure 18.2). The disc may be seen to reduce (recapture) on mouth

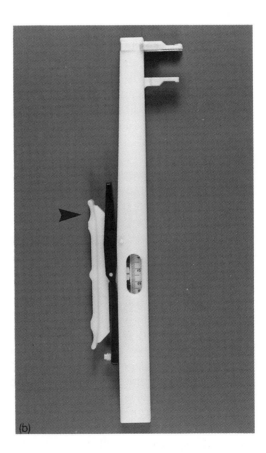
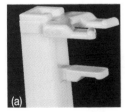

Figure 18.2 Patient-activated positioning device for the TMJ. The patient bites on the upper and lower bite blocks (a) and the bite blocks are widened by the patient pressing on one end of the handle (b) (arrow).

opening (clinically a 'click'), but there are surgical implications for those that do not reduce. It is also important to be able to distinguish normal anatomical variants from pathological problems. Conway et al. (1989) set out to distinguish between the two and found that asymptomatic joints may also show the disc in an anterior position. They suggested that the importance of a pseudo-dynamic technique was, in part, to be able to pinpoint the recapture position of an anteriorly displaced disc in order to decide whether to proceed to surgery or treat the patient conservatively.

Kinematic evaluation of the TMJ should be bilateral (Shellock and Pressman, 1989), as internal derangements are likely to be bilateral. Dual-surface coils reduce the time taken for the examination, and scanning both sides simultaneously enables comparison between the two joints at the same degree of mouth opening; this is important when assessing motion-related abnormalities.

The TMJ condyle is obliqued in both the sagittal and coronal planes and the scanning plane most consistently described is an oblique sagittal positioned from an axial localizer, through the condylar head. The oblique coronal plane may also be useful to visualize medial or lateral displacement of the meniscus (Shellock and Pressman, 1989).

Gradient echo sequences were shown to have some inherent problems, such as magnetic susceptibility, decreased spatial resolution, chemical shift and blood-flow artefacts, but in the cine-loop format gave a good display of joint motion (Burnett et al., 1987). In fact, a variety of sequences are reported for pseudo-dynamic TMJ imaging: T1-weighted spin echo for both static and 'kinematic' studies (Shellock and Pressman, 1989), and T1-weighted spin echo for static open and closed views (Figure 18.3) with gradient echo for the pseudo-dynamic study (Conway et al., 1989). One advantage of gradient echo sequences is the short scan time per incremental position. Using a 25-second gradient echo scan, Conway et al. (1989) experimented with 'active' physiological movement of the jaw, the patient holding their mouth open for 25 seconds in each incremental position. The short scan time eliminates motion artefact, but images have a lower signal-to-noise ratio and lower anatomical resolution. More recently, pseudo-dynamics of the TMJ has been reported by Chen and Buckwalter (1993) who have produced quantitative measurements of condylar displacement. The technique assesses the joint from a fully open to a closed position in 14 increments, an image being taken at each increment, using a jaw positioner with a hydraulic opening system. They characterize condylar motion in this instance, but suggest

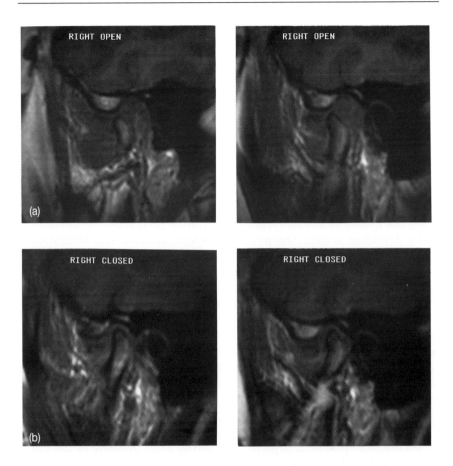

Figure 18.3   Static open (a) and closed (b) views of the TMJ, showing an anteriorly displaced meniscus that does not reduce on mouth opening (T1-weighted spin echo sequence). A dynamic study of this type of abnormality is likely to become a routine part of the TMJ investigation with MRI.

that their quantitative measurements could be applied to the disc motion in future studies.

All the current literature confirms the feasibility of pseudo-dynamic study of the TMJ, but the limitations are associated with being able to capture the speed at which the jaw opens, in a true dynamic study. In the future, the possibility of obtaining ultrafast sequences means that looking at the functional aspects of the joint is likely to become a routine part of the TMJ investigation with MRI.

THE PATELLOFEMORAL JOINT

Applications:
1. Patellar tracking disorders.
2. Anterior knee pain.
3. Chondromalacia.

Clinicians frequently encounter abnormalities of the patellofemoral joint. They are often combined with other lesions and with signs and symptoms that can mimic other knee derangements. The main pathology associated with the joint is malalignment, causing patellar tracking disorders. During knee flexion the patella moves vertically along the groove of the femoral trochlea, with no transverse deviation. If any deviation is seen, the patellar tracking is abnormal. Mechanical divergence from the patellofemoral alignment can cause secondary chondromalacia, damage to articular cartilage or abnormal lateral pressure.

Initially axial projections of the patella were used to measure patellofemoral deviation with the use of angular indices (Merchant et al., 1974; Laurin et al., 1979). However, the technique had its limitations, because projections of the patella could not be obtained at less than 20° flexion. It is now apparent that patellofemoral subluxation is most likely to occur in the first 20° of flexion from extension and that by the time the knee is flexed to 30° or 40° many subluxations have reduced to normal.

Computerized tomography (CT) scanning became the examination of choice for patellofemoral disorders, allowing axial imaging of the knee joint in all positions of flexion, from full flexion to full extension. The use of ultrafast CT scanning gave images that could then be viewed in a cine-loop format. It was this method that identified tracking abnormalities in the 0–20° range of flexion (Delgardo-Martins, 1979).

MRI is the latest imaging technique to be used to evaluate patellar tracking abnormalities but until recently the technique was still only pseudo-dynamic. Shellock et al. (1988) described a technique using T1-weighted spin echo images in the axial plane through the patellofemoral joint. They had designed a positioning device to attach to their table which allowed the patient to lie prone and enabled the knees to flex passively through 0–32° in eight incremental positions. The positioning device was moved to the new position of flexion by the MR operator. A later design (Shellock et al., 1989) modified the apparatus to be activated by a handle operated by the patient (Figure 18.4). In both procedures, ankles and thighs were strapped for immobilization and to

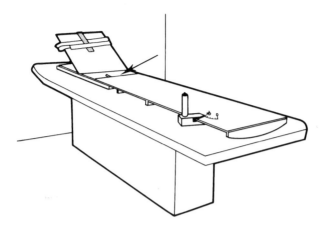

Figure 18.4   Positioning device (Shellock et al., 1989) for pseudo-dynamic MRI of the patellofemoral joints. Note the cut-out portion (arrow) for the knees, freeing them of any external pressure.

stop the legs internally or externally rotating during flexion. A cut-out portion in the device meant that the knees themselves were free of any external pressure. From their work, Shellock et al. (1989) describe four malalignments seen on MR images.

The development of fast-scanning sequences allowed the next development in this technique. Shellock et al. (1991b) used the same positioning device with the cut-out area for the knees, but did not use the activation handle. Instead, the patient began with leg extension and after hearing the scanning sequence start, gradually flexed both joints until their feet touched the inside of the magnet bore. This was termed 'active joint flexion'. The patient practised the technique beforehand to make sure their movement was as even as possible. The scanning sequence used was an ultrafast gradient echo in the axial plane and the flexion procedure was carried out at three different slice locations (through the knee joint) with six sequential images scanned during joint flexion. Images were then displayed in a cine-loop format, and individually.

This technique could now be described as a true 'dynamic' investigation, looking at 'active' movement. Examination time was reduced, influence of muscle contraction could be seen and there was no longer any need for the special positioning device. A further investigation by the same group described active joint flexion against resistance, which was applied to the joint in the sagittal plane using a special positioning device (Shellock et al., 1993). When the joints were flexed under this

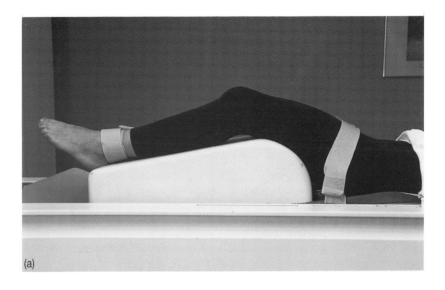

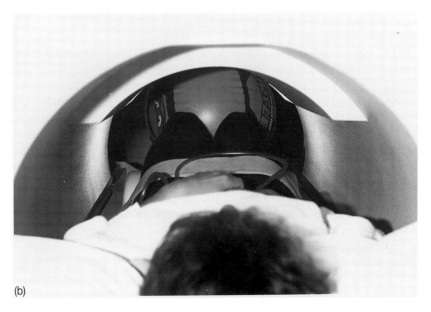

Figure 18.5   Positioning for a dynamic study of the patellofemoral joints: (a) immobilization; (b) patient in position in the magnet bore; (c) position in flexion; (d) position in extension.

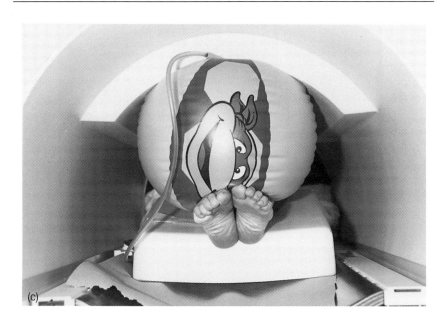

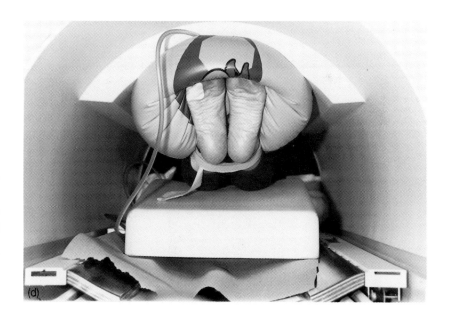

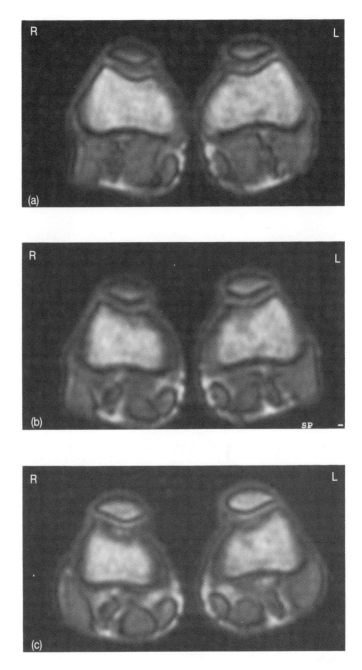

Figure 18.6   (caption opposite)

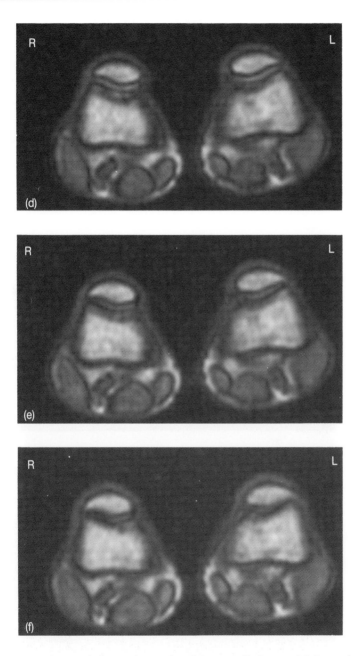

Figure 18.6   Normal dynamic study of the patellofemoral joints, showing flexion (a) to extension (f).

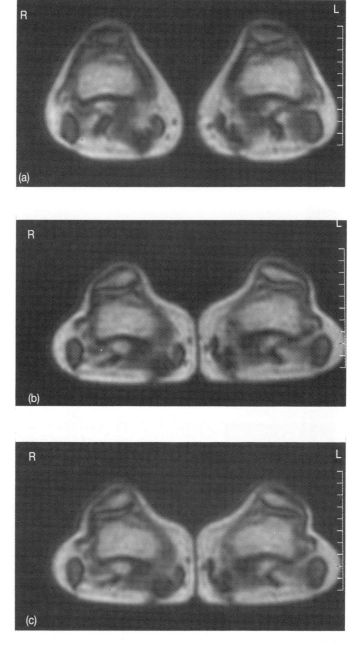

Figure 18.7   (caption opposite)

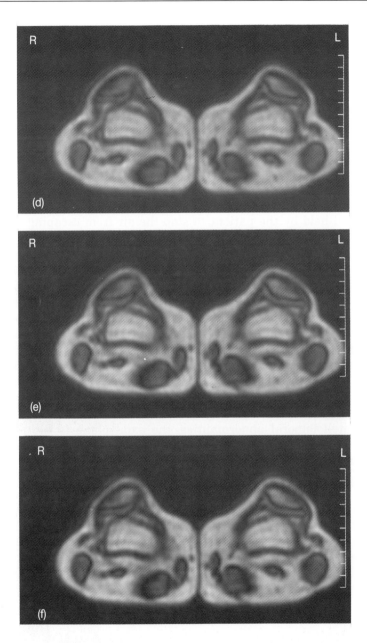

Figure 18.7 Abnormal dynamic study of the patellofemoral joints, showing bilateral patellar subluxation; flexion (a) to extension (f). The lateral retinacula buckle as the patella subluxes.

'loaded' condition, abnormal alignment became more pronounced and some normal alignment on the 'unloaded' study became abnormal on the 'loaded' study. Therefore, there was an increased likelihood of identifying abnormalities in the patellofemoral joint.

A different approach to this dynamic technique, described by P. Emberton and A. Moody (personal communication, 1994) has been adapted in our own department. It requires no special positioning device and seems to identify patellar tracking abnormalities very adequately. The patient lies supine and is immobilized with Velcro straps, with the knees flexed over an angular block (Figure 18.5(a)). A beachball is inflated via a length of tubing, which is inserted into the nozzle of the beachball far enough to break the plastic valve. The tubing is flexed and held by the patient to stop the air from escaping and the beachball is placed over the tibiae of the patient once they have been centralized in the magnet bore (Figure 18.5(b)). The correct slices are located on localizer scans and then an ultrafast gradient echo sequence (Siemens, Turboflash) is used, in the axial and sagittal planes. Multiple sequential images are scanned whilst the patient releases the tube, pushes against the beachball with their legs, forcing it to deflate and hence actively extending their knees (Figure 18.5(c,d)). The scanning stops once the patient indicates that their knees are fully extended. The resulting axial images are run in a cine-loop format to view. The sagittal images are also run in a cine-loop format indicating the angular degree of flexion. Examples of a normal and abnormal study using this technique are shown in Figures 18.6 and 18.7.

For patellofemoral abnormalities, the axial plane is the plane of choice but for internal derangements sagittal pseudo-dynamic studies are useful. The gating system described by Niitsu et al. (1990, 1991) allows passive knee flexion every 2 seconds through the 15–45° range. A small circular coil attached to a knee brace images sagittally while a gradient echo sequence is performed, with slices taken through the intercondylar notch. Comparison with static three-dimensional MRI reveals increased sensitivity and specificity for anterior cruciate ligament tears and there is better assessment of the cruciates generally, particularly their 'tightness'. Movement of free fragments of meniscus (not seen on static MRI) is also well visualized.

CONCLUSION

Although the techniques of dynamic scanning of most joints are in their early stages, those for the TMJ and patellofemoral joints are the most promising and clinically useful to date. The full potential of the dynamic technique is yet to be realized. Having developed their technique, Shellock et al. (1994) have gone on to evaluate a 'patellar realignment brace' using their 'loaded' study. This may point to the future of dynamic techniques in therapeutic assessment.

As far as the technique itself is concerned, the more 'real-time' the procedure can be, the better. This suggests that development of faster sequences such as echo planar sequences must play an increasingly important role in the future.

References

Bonutti, P.M., Norfray, J.F., Friedman, R.J. et al. (1993) Technical note: kinematic MRI of the shoulder. *Journal of Computer Assisted Tomography* **17:** 666–669.

Burnett, K.R., Davis, C.L., Read, J. (1987) Dynamic display of the temporomandibular joint meniscus by using 'fast-scan' MR imaging. *American Journal of Roentgenology* **149:** 959–962.

Chen, J., Buckwalter, K. (1993) Displacement analysis of the temporomandibular condyle from magnetic resonance images. *Journal of Biomechanics* **26:** 1455–1462.

Conway, W.F., Hayes, C.W., Campbell, R.L. et al. (1989) Temporomandibular joint motion: efficacy of fast low angle shot MR imaging. *Radiology* **172:** 821–826.

Delgago-Martins, H. (1979) A study of the position of the patella using computerised tomography. *Journal of Bone and Joint Surgery* **61:** 443–444.

Kawaida, H., Takashi, S., Yoshiyuki, M. et al. (1989) Magnetic resonance imaging of upper cervical disorders in rheumatoid arthritis. *Spine* **14:** 1144–1148.

Laurin, C.A. Dussault, R., Levesque, H.P. (1979) The tangential x-ray investigation of the patellofemoral joint: x-ray technique, diagnostic criteria and their interpretation. *Clinical Orthopaedics* **144:** 16–26.

McAfee, P.C., Bohlman, H.H., Hans, J.S. et al. (1986) Comparison of nuclear magnetic resonance imaging and computed tomography in the diagnosis of upper cervical spine cord compression. *Spine* **11:** 295–304.

Merchant, A.C., Mercer, R.L., Jacobsen, R.H. et al. (1974) Roentgenographic analysis of patellofemoral congruence. *Journal of Bone and Joint Surgery* **56A:** 1391–1396.

Niitsu, M., Akisada, M., Anno, I. et al. (1990) Moving knee joint: technique for kinematic MR imaging. *Radiology* **174:** 569–570.

Niitsu, M., Anno, I., Fukabayashi, T. et al. (1991) Tears of cruciate ligaments and menisci: evaluation with cine MR imaging. *Radiology* **178:** 859–864.

Olerud, C., Kongsholm, J., Thuomas, K.A. (1988) The congruence of the distal radioulnar joint. A magnetic resonance imaging study. *Acta Orthopaedica Scandinavica* **59:** 183–185.

Shellock, F.G., Pressman, B.D. (1989) Dual-surface-coil MR imaging of bilateral temporomandibular joints: improvements in the imaging protocol. *American Journal of Neuroradiology* **10:** 595–598.

Shellock, F.G., Mink, J.H., Fox, J.M. (1988) Patellofemoral joint: kinematic MR imaging to assess tracking abnormalities. *Radiology* **168:** 551–553.

Shellock, F.G., Mink, J.H., Deutsch, A. et al. (1989) Patellar tracking abnormalities: clinical experience with kinematic MR imaging in patients. *Radiology* **172:** 799–804.

Shellock, F.G., Mink, J.H., Deutsch, A. et al. (1991a) Kinematic magnetic resonance imaging of the joints: techniques and clinical applications. *Magnetic Resonance Quarterly* **7:** 104–135.

Shellock, F.G., Foo, T.K.F., Deutsch, A. et al. (1991b) Patellofemoral joint: evaluation during active flexion with ultrafast spoiled GRASS MR imaging. *Radiology* **180:** 581–585.

Shellock, F.G., Mink, J.H., Deutsch, A.L. et al. (1993) Patellofemoral joint: identification of abnormalities with active-movement. 'Unloaded' versus 'loaded' kinematic MR imaging techniques. *Radiology* **188:** 575–578.

Shellock, F.G., Mink, J.H., Deutsch, A.L. et al. (1994) Effect of a patellar realignment brace on patellofemoral relationships: evaluation with kinematic MR imaging. *Journal of Magnetic Resonance Imaging* **4:** 590–594.

Skie, M., Zeiss, J., Ebraham, N.A. et al. (1990) Carpal tunnel changes and median nerve compression during wrist flexion and extension seen by magnetic resonance imaging. *Journal of Hand Surgery* **15A:** 934–939.

Yoshioka, S., Okuda., Y., Tamai, K. et al. (1993) Changes in carpal tunnel shape during wrist joint motion. MRI evaluation of normal volunteers. *Journal of Hand Surgery (British and European Volume)* **18B:** 620–623.

19

Spiral Computed Tomography: Current Applications and Future Potential

Leonie S. Paskin

INTRODUCTION

It was time for a new development in computed tomography (CT) scanning:

- to give potential customers a sound technological reason to replace older scanners, the market for new ones having reached, virtually, saturation point.
- to enable radiologists to keep at bay the threat from magnetic resonance imaging (MRI) and to retain a major role for CT in cross-sectional imaging.
- to decrease the daily stress for radiographers in many CT units caused by waiting lists considered to be too long and the ever-present need to increase daily throughput.
- for patients who needed CT to be more available and accessible, to be a better tool for diagnosis and management, and to give their clinicians an aid to planning for all eventualities.

All major X-ray equipment manufacturers now have on the market CT scanners capable of volume acquisition, the performance of some of which outshines others. The movement used for large-volume acquisition is commonly called 'spiral', but is sometimes known as 'helical' or even 'double-helical' scanning – the exact movement being determined by each manufacturer.

DEVELOPMENT

The basic physics of spiral CT does not differ from that of conventional CT. The development that was to prove crucial to longer, faster scanning was an innovation in gantry technology and design – the slip ring. The continuous circular movement of the data-acquisition system and continuous table movement is the main distinguishing feature between volume scanning and conventional scanning.

Slip-ring technology is now based in third- and fourth-generation scanners. This technology means that the power is transferred by two rings slipping against each other. The outer ring houses both the tube and the detectors, with brushes attached to it. The brushes make contact with an inner metallic ring which is connected directly to a generator. This means that rotations can continue indefinitely in one direction: there are now no cables to be pulled taut and to be wound and rewound, one of the major limiting factors in rotations for conventional CT. It should be noted that slip-ring technology can be used even when spiral scanning is not needed and that most scanners would be used in both spiral and conventional modes.

To cope with volume scanning demands and future demands based on the slip-ring innovation, two other major CT components had to be updated and modified. Tubes had to be able to bear a high heat capacity and/or have rapid cooling mechanisms to allow for long, continuous exposure. Tables had to be modified for continuous, accurate and smooth incrementation. On the software side, work needed to be done on the image data processing to minimize degradation of image quality that would occur due to the continual movement of tube and patient. This still remains one of the most difficult problems to be overcome, but to some manufacturers' credit it is often extremely difficult to distinguish an image taken in spiral mode from a conventional image.

GENERAL BENEFITS OF VOLUME ACQUISITION

Spiral scanning has provided the ability to cut the scanning time dramatically. On the highest specification scanner it is possible to scan from the apices of the lungs to the symphysis pubis in 60 seconds (provided that patients can hold their breath). When a complete block of tissue is imaged in one breathhold nothing is missed, as in conventional scanning, because of the variation in respiratory pattern. As a result, objective evaluation of diseases and responses of diseases to treatment is vastly improved, as is the degree of anatomical detail displayed, which helps with complex surgery.

The need for anaesthetic and sedation in CT has greatly diminished due to the speed of scanning time. Patients brought to CT from intensive therapy units (ITUs) should spend less time away from their stable environment. In some instances CT has replaced more invasive diagnostic imaging examinations such as angiography and barium enemas.

It must, however, be pointed out that volume scanning in itself is not a method which will increase patient throughput. It is usually slower on the image-processing side than conventional scanning, especially if radiologists insist on 'playing' with the many processing options available. Currently, there is associated progress to make conventional scanning faster and so, in general, using a mix of spiral and conventional CT more patients per day can be scanned and waiting lists can be cut.

Volume scanning, that is the ability to scan continuously with nothing other than physiological movement to mar the image, makes three-dimensional reconstructions and sagittal and coronal reformats superior. All this can be achieved with similar radiation doses to those used in conventional CT.

DISADVANTAGES OF VOLUME SCANNING

Volume scanning is slower in the varied reconstruction phases than is conventional CT, because blocks of tissue can often be reconstructed at varying intervals. High heat loading is placed on the tube, adding to its wear and tear. On some scanners image quality is significantly degraded, but this is an area for continued research and development.

Patients can find it difficult to hold their breath for long periods of time. Adequate coaching and preparation using hyperventilation techniques mean the greatest benefits can be achieved by this method of scanning.

CLINICAL IMPLICATIONS

It is now possible to tailor-make protocols for clinical conditions. The parameters that are operator-selective are exposure factors, length of exposure, slice thickness, reconstruction algorithm and newest reconstruction increment, so making it possible to reconstruct a slice of a predetermined thickness anywhere along a block of tissue. The slice thickness is set at the time of scanning and cannot be altered subsequently. However, it is possible to reconstruct at any interval along the tissue volume. It is also possible to produce reconstructed overlapping slices with no increase in radiation dose.

CLINICAL APPLICATIONS

It is accepted that spiral CT has brought an older imaging modality back to state of the art. It is claiming new territory from angiography and plain-film radiology and is regaining some of the ground lost to MRI.

There has been much discussion as to whether spiral scanning contributes directly to lower contrast agent use per procedure. Faster scanning certainly allows optimum tracking of a single bolus injection of contrast agent and lower iodine strengths can be used. However, it is a great temptation to give contrast agent in cases where previously it would not have been used. It is essential to have a contrast agent injector to make best use of spiral CT so that delivery of the contrast agent can be accurately timed and examinations can be consistently repeated.

The Brain and Nervous System

MRI continues to provide superior diagnostic imaging in this field. Some work is currently being done on spiral CT of the circle of Willis. Spiral CT is also likely to fill in the gaps that MRI leaves; for example, patients who cannot tolerate MRI or who for various reasons cannot be subjected to a magnetic field.

The Neck

Swallowing has always caused motion artefact when scanning the neck structures. This problem is virtually eliminated by the speed of spiral CT. Narrow interval reconstructions provide superb anatomical detail of vessels and adjacent structures (Figure 19.1). This is an area where the use of spiral CT will yield diagnostic images, while conventional CT would have failed, most especially if the patient's airway was compromised and speed was an essential element.

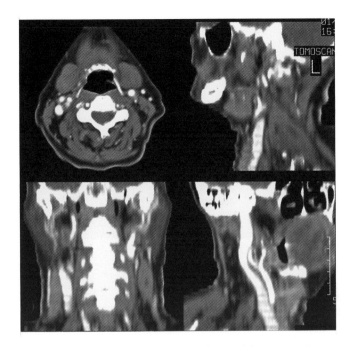

Figure 19.1 Oblique reformatted image showing normal carotid bifurcation.

The Chest

Spiral CT allows the whole chest to be imaged in a single breathhold. Small lesions now have a greater chance of detection and the anatomical detail of the bronchial airways is unsurpassed. The physiological movement of the heart has always marred image quality, and spiral CT helps overcome this problem. Superior imaging is an important aid to planning the management and treatment of any chest problem and, once again, the speed element can be very important to the breathless patient requiring a chest scan.

The Abdomen

CT has always been used widely to image all abdominal pathology. Spiral CT offers an improvement in early detection of abdominal disease (Figure 19.2). A rapid delivery of a bolus of contrast agent followed

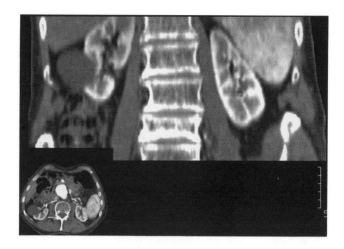

Figure 19.2   Coronal, reformatted image showing renal cyst.

by fast data acquisition showing peaks of contrast enhancement in any particular organ is an essential element.

CT of the abdomen has always presented certain problems, particularly with regard to how to differentiate between various types of tissue. Thin slices, rapid scanning and timed, accurate delivery of contrast agent can help to accentuate the tissue differences. Small lesions detected early can have an impact on the patient's prognosis and quality of life.

In the liver, tumours are highly vascular and the extent of invasion can be clearly seen. Many, but not all, liver metastases are hypovascular. Sometimes this subtle difference in imaging patterns can help in the search for the primary tumour.

In the pancreas, a question of whether disease is malignant or benign can arise. Spiral CT offers the ability to distinguish a neoplasm from pancreatitis (although this is not always easy) by looking at contrast agent enhancement patterns. Necrosis or haemorrhage within the organ can be assessed, as can invasion of disease into neighbouring organs or vessels.

Conventional CT of the kidney has often been suboptimal, mainly due to respiratory motion and the partial volume effect. Both these problems are virtually eliminated when spiral CT is used. The entire kidney can be imaged in one breathhold. Examining the kidney at times of peak enhancement improves the ability to distinguish between renal masses and parenchymal disease (Figure 19.3). Delayed

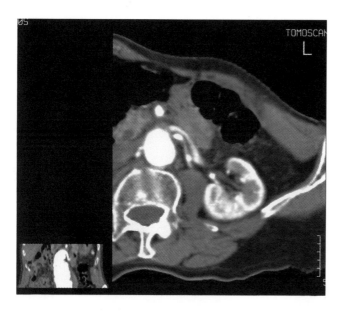

Figure 19.3   Transaxial image of renal artery, coming off just above aortic aneurysm.

scans can also be very helpful, as an area for error previously has been venous infiltration of renal tumours. To help determine if the inferior vena cava is involved, as well as the renal vein, three-dimensional reconstructions can be made using artefact-free spiral data.

FRACTURES AND BONE WORK

Spiral CT and its associated reformats and reconstructions are of great value to orthopaedic surgeons. In acute trauma situations, data can be acquired quickly and high-quality images are available rapidly so the best surgical option for patients can be determined (Figure 19.4). Precise information about fractures and placements of tiny bony fragments is vital. Maximum length spiral CT scans, up to 60 cm, can be employed if necessary, as often breathholding is not needed.

Three-dimensional reconstructions have proved very valuable to faciomaxillary surgeons in trauma cases and in facial anomaly cases, especially as low-dose spiral scanning has been developed for facial work.

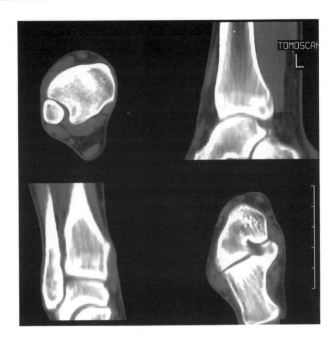

Figure 19.4   Transaxial, coronal and sagittal image of a normal ankle, showing the bone and the soft-tissue component.

It is worth making the point at this stage that, although many scanners are multitasking and can do much of the work in the background, if much work needs three-dimensional construction and multiplanar reformats, a separate workstation needs to be available. This allows radiologists and clinicians the opportunity to 'play' with images without holding up scanning lists.

CT ANGIOGRAPHY

If a CT scanner, capable of very fast data acquisition, is to carry out angiographic-type examinations the contrast agent must be administered rapidly, steadily and consistently. The differing hand-injection strengths of radiologists were not too much of a problem when conventional CT was used but if spiral CT is to be used to perform scans to investigate vascular problems, a reliable contrast-agent injector is a prerequisite.

Conventional angiography is not without risk and non-invasive tests that can replace it should be used. Spiral CT is particularly good for imaging dissection and aneurysm of the thoracic and abdominal aorta; again, its speed is particularly helpful in the acute situation (Figure 19.5). The size and extent of the aneurysm can be delineated, and its relationship to other vessels and intimal flaps can be clearly seen. The renal arteries can also be well visualized, as can other specifically targeted abdominal vessels. It is unlikely, however, that spiral CT will offer much benefit in the imaging of peripheral vascular disease other than, possibly, in targeting certain vessels.

CT INTERVENTION

Spiral CT can make guided biopsies and drainage of fluid collections easier. Short spiral sequences obtained during a single breathhold can be used to determine needle and catheter-tip placement with great

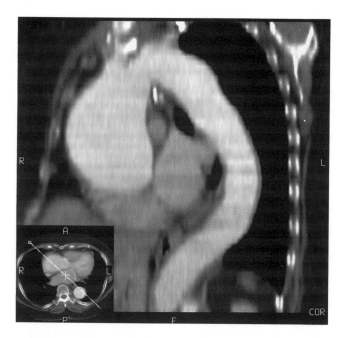

Figure 19.5 Sagittal reformat of a large ascending aortic aneurysm and a tortuous descending aorta.

accuracy, which makes the examination less traumatic for the patient. Follow-up can also be achieved rapidly and comfortably, in conjunction with repositioning of a drainage tube if necessary. Where interventional work forms a large part of the workload it should be remembered that *only* the scanning time is shorter; everything else takes the same amount of time as it did with conventional CT.

PROTOCOLS

Protocols for spiral CT scanning are important and should be driven by radiologists who know the capabilities of the scanner and have the relevant medical knowledge.

It is important to follow protocols developed for particular clinical conditions, especially where the staff in a CT unit are not permanent but are rotational. This is particularly so if volume scanning is often used. It is too easy and tempting to do short spiral sequences that take no time at all but yield only additional radiation dose and no better diagnostic information. It is essential to understand in both pathological and physiological terms what needs to be demonstrated. Radiologists and radiographers need to work as a team to set up the protocols and ensure they are adhered to. Where this is appreciated, a better working environment for all and a higher patient throughout are the results.

CONCLUSIONS

Volumetric scanning offers considerable advantages over conventional CT. The continual rotation adds new items of information to the data that were previously available. This offers significant advantages to the referring clinicians in the decision-making and the treatment-management processes. Difficult examinations have become far more tolerable to patients and, in some cases, spiral CT has replaced invasive diagnostic tests which carried known risks. Has spiral CT saved the CT radiologist and radiographer? Maybe, for a year or two.

Spiral CT scanning does impact on everyday life in CT units. It is now necessary for radiographers to get to grips with physiology, as well as anatomy, as the physiology affects how the scan is carried out and because radiographers are able to influence the images that the scanner produces.

WHAT NEXT?

Since the introduction of volume scanning, much work has been done by the manufacturers of X-ray tubes to enable them to produce high-rated exposures without delays for the cooling process. The reconstruction algorithms have been improved almost to the point where it is difficult, even to a trained eye, to distinguish between slices of transpiral CT and those taken in the conventional way. The post-processing software for multiplanar and three-dimensional reconstruction continues to improve, but work needs to continue in this field, as it does in the area of computer capacity, because so many patients are amenable to spiral scanning.

It is said 'It is a fact that in these times the computer is an indispensable tool in the creation of a medical image, it is the computer that brings the image to life. The medical questions remain the same but the new visual tool chest answers them faster and more efficiently' (Zonneveld, 1992). The future developments for spiral CT are in the minds of doctors and scientists and the hands of manufacturers. What next?

Acknowledgements

I would like to include my thanks to Dr Sheila Rankin for making the introduction of spiral CT into our department as smooth and easy as possible and for her never-ending efforts to keep our protocols updated. Thanks also to Philips Medical Systems for their help and guidance. All illustrations are from the Philips SR 7000 Volumetric CT Scanner.

References

Zonneveld, F.W. (1992) Inaugural lecture on becoming Professor of Medical Imaging Techniques. Utrecht: University of Utrecht.

20

Perfusion Computed Tomography

Vivian Wood

INTRODUCTION

Computerized tomography (CT) is acknowledged universally as an essential method of describing anatomical detail and the way in which it is altered by disease processes. Its value as a method of functional imaging has only been acknowledged recently.

Perfusion CT is a method of producing a quantifiable map of contrast-medium uptake within a volume of tissue and applying a colour scale to represent varying degrees of perfusion, in the same way that a grey scale is used to represent varying CT attenuation values.

Until now, absolute measurement of tissue perfusion has relied on nuclear medicine techniques or intra-arterial gas washout, the latter being a highly invasive procedure. The advantages of CT over nuclear medicine are shown in Table 20.1.

CT perfusion studies can often be arranged to coincide with a diagnostic examination being undertaken for reasons related to the patient's disease. The procedure becomes a small addition to the examination, additional doses of contrast medium and radiation are minimized and the increase in overall examination time is negligible.

The colour plate section for this article appears between p. 244 and p. 245.

Table 20.1 The advantages of CT

	Nuclear medicine
ion of blood volume of tissue l by the area of interest and the ss	More difficult to achieve. The procedure becomes more invasive
tional imaging atial resolution	Limited by the resolving capacity of the gamma camera
resolution. n acquire data d intervals. olume-acquisition ire at 1-second reconstruct at ntervals	Can also acquire counts at 1-second intervals
ration within an e measured; 25 nits is equivalent concentration of iles et al., 1991). refore, a linear between iodine CT attenuation	Not applicable
invasive – e delivery of unt of contrast an intravenous	Relatively non-invasive in the simplest form of the procedure

JE

re involves the rapid acquisition of a series of scan data at tomical level after the delivery of a bolus of contrast gions of interest (ROIs) are then drawn within or around ssels of interest within each scan section of the sequence. Time-density curves (TDCs) are generated for each series of ROIs. These measure tissue perfusion by adapting data-processing techniques used in nuclear medicine studies to quantify temporal changes in density within the chosen ROI (Peters et al., 1987a,b). This is made possible by the fact that radiographic contrast media have similar pharmacokinetics to radiopharmaceuticals. The precise details of the procedure will vary between centres, particularly with regard to the amount of contrast agent, rate of delivery and timing of data acquisition, but the sequence of events remains constant.

DATA ANALYSIS

Tissue perfusion is defined as flow per unit volume. Mullani and Gould (1983) developed the most widely used algorithm for calculating perfusion in the myocardium. The perfusion is given by the ratio of the maximal tissue-density increase to the area under the curve, after correction for recirculation.

$$\text{Perfusion} = \frac{F}{V}$$

where F is the flow and V is the volume of tissue sampled. Perfusion is measured in millilitres per minute per millilitre.

Miles et al. (1991) were the first authors to describe perfusion CT. They used CT data to generate a quantifiable map of tissue perfusion displayed by means of a colour scale. The colour scale extended from dark blue representing $0\,\text{ml}\,\text{min}^{-1}\text{ml}^{-1}$, through blue-green up to $2\,\text{ml}\,\text{min}^{-1}\text{ml}^{-1}$, green-yellow up to $3\,\text{ml}\,\text{min}^{-1}\text{ml}^{-1}$ and red-pink-white, with white representing $5\,\text{ml}\,\text{min}^{-1}\text{ml}^{-1}$. The image and colour scale were displayed together, enabling absolute perfusion to be read (Plates 1–3).

Blomley, M.J.K., Coulden, R., Dawson, P. and co workers (unpublished data, 1994) adapted the perfusion formula further and related it directly to CT to give:

$$\text{Perfusion} = \frac{\text{Peak rise in parenchymal CT no.}}{\text{Area under aortic time attenuation curve}}$$

The peak rise in parenchymal CT number is expressed in hounsfield units and the area under the aortic curve in hounsfield unit seconds.

One of the problems inherent in measuring temporal changes in contrast density within living tissue is that, after the first pass around the system, the effects of recirculation are included in the density changes within the tissue in question. In graphical representations this is seen as an initial peak followed by a succession of smaller peaks which represent recirculation of the contrast. Recirculation is eliminated from the time–density curve by the application of a mathematical tool – the gamma variate fit. This is an accepted method of extracting the initial phase from the time–concentration curve of a tracer (Thompson et al., 1963).

Although the mathematical techniques have been successfully applied to data acquired on relatively slow CT scanners, it was the advent of the increased data-acquisition capabilities of continuous-rotation CT equipment which prompted an increased awareness of the potential role of CT in functional imaging techniques. With this type of equipment 1-second exposures are routine, compared with exposure times of 5–20 seconds on older, conventional translate/rotate equipment. The increased speed of continuous rotation machines afforded researchers the luxury of rapid acquisition of data, which is particularly important in the early stage of bolus delivery, i.e. in the first 20 seconds. This is where the rate of change of arterial enhancement is most rapid and is unaffected by recirculation. Once the venous phase of the injection becomes apparent and recirculation begins to contribute to appearances of enhancement, rapid data-acquisition becomes less important and scan rate can be reduced from one per second to one every 5 seconds.

Despite the recent advances in CT hardware, on-line software packages are still somewhat primitive in their ability to undertake the type of evaluation required to produce functional information. For this reason it is common to download the data to an independent terminal and use alternative, off-line software to do the analysis and colour encoding. This has the advantage of not interrupting the daily flow of work and is an important consideration as this part of the study can be time consuming. Those centres which already undertake similar analysis of data acquired from magnetic resonance imaging (MRI) and positron emission tomography (PET) usually have access to suitable software. As the role of CT perfusion develops and becomes established in clinical use, on-line software will undoubtedly be developed to meet the need.

APPLICATIONS

This section discusses some of the work done to date, as a means of demonstrating the potential of the technique. It is not, however, an exhaustive or comprehensive summary of the applications of the technique. Much of the work undertaken to date originates from the

Hammersmith and Addenbrooke's hospitals in the UK, and the University of Chicago Hospital, USA. Between them these centres have measured perfusion in the chest, liver, kidneys, pancreas, spleen and brain.

The Liver

Measurement of liver perfusion is complicated by the biphasic nature of its blood supply. Contrast medium arrives first via the hepatic arterial supply and slightly later via the hepatic portal system.

Nuclear medicine perfusion studies have proven valuable in studying patients with liver metastases, cirrhosis and in evaluating patients who have undergone liver transplantation. Functional images of hepatic blood flow have also been produced, but the resolution has been poor and evaluation is limited to the right lobe only, due to overlap of the inferior vena cava and aorta on the left lobe giving an exaggerated impression of vascular activity within the left lobe.

The original short report by Miles et al. (1991) was followed by a study, again by Miles et al. (1993), which sought to separate and quantify hepatic arterial and portal perfusion and to display the two components as a ratio – the hepatic perfusion index (HPI). The patients involved were all undergoing dynamic CT of the liver as part of an assessment of known or suspected liver disease. Amongst the abnormal scans were a variety of pathologies, including cirrhosis, primary tumours and metastases.

A scan level was selected which included an area of focal abnormality or, in patients with diffuse liver disease, a level was selected which included the left and the right lobes of the liver as well as the spleen. The following scan sequence was carried out at this level: 1-second acquisition at 0, 7, 10, 13, 16, 21, 26, 31, 37.5 and 44 seconds after the injection of contrast medium. Time–density curves were generated from circular ROIs drawn over the aorta, the right lobe of liver, the left lobe of liver and the spleen. Values for arterial and portal perfusion were used to produce the HPI according to the equation:

$$HPI = \frac{\text{Arterial perfusion}}{\text{Arterial perfusion + Portal perfusion}} \times 100\%$$

All of the diseased livers displayed perfusion values which varied from values for normal livers. In cirrhosis, portal perfusion was reduced due to portal hypertension; however, a compensatory mechanism exists which increases arterial perfusion. In all other groups arterial perfusion was altered to a far greater extent than was portal perfusion. The greatest increase in arterial perfusion was measured in hepatocellular carcinoma. Arterial perfusion was also raised in metastases, but over a much wider range. All liver tumours, whether primary or secondary, derive almost all of their blood supply from the arterial rather than the portal circulation. However, the range of values derived in metastases indicates that the nature of the primary tumour may influence the change in arterial perfusion.

More recently, liver perfusion has been the subject of a study carried out in Chicago (Blomley, M.J.K., Coulden, R., Dawson, P. and co-workers, unpublished data, 1994), using ultrafast CT on an Imatron C100 machine. This allows subsecond scan times and a high repetition rate; for example, one study involved the acquisition of 20–40 scans of 0.4- or 0.1-second duration. The high temporal resolution of the system increases the accuracy of the calculations.

Liver studies sought to provide absolute quantification of hepatic arterial and portal venous perfusion. The methods for deriving all the values differed from those used by the previous authors. It should be noted, however, that whilst the two groups of authors may not agree on methods of data analysis, they do seem to have reached the same conclusions, if not the same absolute values. A value of $0.19\,\mathrm{ml\,min^{-1}ml^{-1}}$ was reached for normal arterial perfusion. This was elevated to $0.25\,\mathrm{ml\,min^{-1}ml^{-1}}$ in cirrhosis and raised further in metastases to $0.43\,\mathrm{ml\,min^{-1}ml^{-1}}$. Normal portal perfusion was found to be $0.93\,\mathrm{ml\,min^{-1}ml^{-1}}$, which reduced to $0.43\,\mathrm{ml\,min^{-1}ml^{-1}}$ in cirrhosis.

The authors concluded that there was scope for this technique to be applied to normal and deranged physiology of the liver, including cirrhosis and tumour circulation. It would also enable the effect of various therapeutic procedures to be evaluated and monitored over an extended period by a relatively non-invasive technique. Such procedures could include the effect of chemotherapy and radiotherapy on tumours, shunting in cases of portal hypertension, interventional radiological procedures such as tumour embolization and transjugular intrahepatic portosystemic shunting. They also concluded that there was potential for the technique to be applied to other cross-sectional imaging modalities. It is likely that in the future MRI and PET will also have significant roles to play in perfusion imaging.

The Spleen

Splenic blood flow is an area which remains incompletely understood and has been evaluated by workers in Chicago, (Blomley, M.J.K.,

Kormano, M., Coulden, R. and coworkers, unpublished data, 1994), again using an Imatron C100. During CT examinations of the abdomen, it is often observed that the spleen enhances patchily, displaying areas of inhomogeneity. This pattern of enhancement is also seen in contrast-enhanced rapid MRI of the liver. It can be a normal appearance in the spleen, but is not found in any other organ, except where disease is present. Values were derived for normal and abnormal splenic perfusion which correlated well with values obtained from intra-arterial xenon washout. Perfusion is reduced in portal hypertension and considerably raised when splenic metastases are present.

The study also investigated the phenomenon of patchy enhancement and found that in all subjects it was a temporary appearance, uniform enhancement being observed 1–2 minutes after injection. It is thought to reflect the nature of the splenic microcirculation, where blood passes first through the white pulp and then through the red pulp, the latter making up most of the splenic parenchyma. Contrast is thought to pass more rapidly through the white pulp than it does through the red pulp, and this probably accounts for the appearances displayed in enhanced CT and MRI studies.

The Kidney

Quantification of the nephrogram and recognizing the ways in which it is affected in disease may be important in the early diagnosis and treatment of conditions such as chronic glomerular disease, acute obstruction, and acute tubular necrosis. Dynamic renal CT and the appropriate data analysis were found to be valuable in demonstrating the distribution of contrast medium within the kidney. Dawson and Peters (1994) studied three patients, all of whom were undergoing CT examination during the treatment of malignant disease. A midkidney section was located from the diagnostic scan, a 40-ml bolus was then delivered by injection pump at $5 \, \text{ml s}^{-1}$. The acquisition sequence was initiated after 20 ml of the bolus had been delivered, and scans were taken every 5 seconds for 2 minutes. ROIs were drawn first around the whole kidney and then within the aorta to generate arterial/aortic and renogram time–density curves. The curves generated clearly demonstrated the dynamics of the physiology of the kidneys and the way in which contrast is handled within the kidney. With refinement and the quantification of normal limits of function, there is potential for the technique to be applied to those situations where an abnormal nephrogram is a significant indication of renal disease, both in the acute and chronic phases, and transplant rejection.

CONCLUSION

From the work discussed above, it is becoming apparent that CT has a very valuable role to play in functional imaging. This holds true despite the fact much of the work is still in its infancy and authors do not necessarily agree as yet on a standard technique.

Acknowledgements

I am extremely grateful to the following people for their invaluable assistance with this chapter: Dr Martin Blomley, who allowed access to his work, much of which has yet to be published; Dr Kenneth Miles, who also gave access to his work and supplied the illustrations; Ms Tracy Tighe, for secretarial support; and Mr John Laird, for proofreading and constructive comments.

References

Dawson, P., Peters, A.M. (1994) What is the nephrogram? *British Journal of Radiology* **67:** 21–25.

Miles, K.A., Hayball, M., Dixon, A.K. (1991) Colour perfusion imaging: a new application of computed tomography. *Lancet* **337:** 643–645.

Miles, K.A., Hayball, M., Dixon, A.K. (1993) Functional images of hepatic perfusion with dynamic CT. *Radiology* **188:** 405–411.

Mullani, N.J., Gould, R.J. (1983) First pass measurements of regional blood flow using external detectors. *Journal of Nuclear Medicine* **24:** 577–581.

Peters, A.M., Brown, J., Hartnell, G.G. et al. (1987a) Non-invasive measurement of renal blood flow with ^{99m}Tc DTPA: a comparison with radiolabelled microspheres. *Cardiovascular Research* **21:** 830–834.

Peters, A.M., Gunasekera, R.D., Henderson, B.L. et al. (1987b) Non-invasive measurements of blood flow and extraction fraction. *Nuclear Medicine Communications* **8:** 823–837.

Thompson, H.K., Starmer, C.F., Whalen, R.E. et al. (1963) Indicator transit time considered as a gamma variate. *Circulation Research* **14:** 502–515.

21

Positron Emission Tomography – A Clinical Tool?

John Lowe

PRINCIPLES OF POSITRON EMISSION TOMOGRAPHY

Positron emission tomography (PET) is a radiotracer technique which utilizes the positron emitting radionuclides oxygen-15, carbon-11, nitrogen-13 and fluorine-18. These can be readily incorporated into bio-molecules. Because of their short half-lives and the high specific activities produced, it is possible to perform serial studies in vivo using amounts of radiotracer which will not alter the physiology of the system under investigation.

The radionuclides are produced in a cyclotron (Figure 21.1). This works by accelerating a beam of charged particles in a circular motion and bombarding a target, chosen to produce a specific radionuclide. Some positron-emitting tracers such as [^{13}N]-ammonia (^{13}NH$_3$) are produced directly in the target, while others are produced by means of appropriate chemical reactions; for example, [^{18}F]fluorodeoxyglucose (^{18}FDG) and ^{11}C-methionine.

Hundreds of tracer substances have been synthesized, but the majority of clinical PET studies worldwide are carried out using the glucose analogue ^{18}FDG. This plays an important role in clinical work as it allows visualization of glucose metabolism. The advantage of this glucose analogue is that it is trapped at a known stage in the metabolic pathway. This trapping and its 110-minute half-life make it practical for clinical imaging over a period of minutes or hours. Other positron-

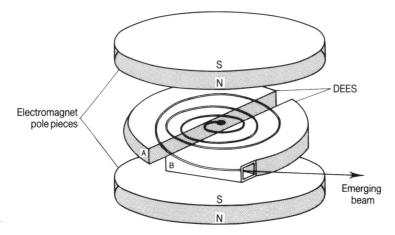

A and B represent entry points for alternating voltage supply

Figure 21.1 Diagram to illustrate principle of the cyclotron.

emitting tracers useful in clinical work include $^{13}NH_3$ used to assess cardiac perfusion, [^{11}C]methionine used to visualize tumours and $H_2{}^{15}O$ to image brain perfusion.

Positron emissions are detected in vivo by means of a radial array of detectors surrounding a patient (Figure 21.2). A positron travels a distance of a few millimetres in tissue before annihilating with an electron, causing two γ photons to be emitted at 180° to one another. The detectors work in coincidence to map the lines of response of each annihilation event. These data are manipulated by computer and back-projected to produce transaxial tomographic images.

In a modern machine spatial resolution is approximately 5 mm full width at half maximum (Spinks et al., 1988). A correction for attenuation at depth is performed using a positron-emitting source rotated around the patient before the emission study. PET can provide quantitative information in absolute terms, for example blood flow in millilitres per minute per gram, but this may require arterial blood sampling as well as serial measurements of metabolite levels during a study.

LOGISTICS OF CLINICAL PET

A cyclotron and radiochemistry laboratory are needed to produce positron-emitting tracers. The cyclotron must be shielded and sited in

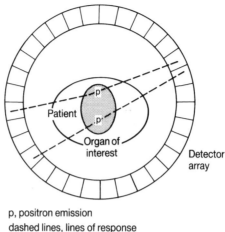

p, positron emission
dashed lines, lines of response

Figure 21.2   Schematic diagram to illustrate principle of PET imaging.

a basement with all necessary safety measures. Negative-ion cyclotrons are favoured because it is possible to split the beam to bombard two targets simultaneously. Automated radiochemistry apparatus may save on staff costs as well as reducing radiation dosage to personnel. Radionuclides may be pumped from one location to another along fine-bore piping, and on-line quality control apparatus such as liquid chromatography is needed to ensure radiochemical purity. A scanner and computer are needed to acquire and process images. Several skilled staff, including a radiographer, a physicist, a chemist and a cyclotron technician, are needed to operate and maintain the machinery.

Where transport links are good, it may be possible to use the relatively longer lived PET tracers, for example [18]FDG, at a remote location. As a rule of thumb, this may be possible where the travelling time is less than one half-life of the desired radionuclide. A large centre with a cyclotron may thereby supply several sites which do not possess the expensive synthesis apparatus. A shift system for radiotracer production and scanner operation may reduce unit costs per study.

Commercial companies are trying to make use of cheaper technology for PET scanning apparatus. There is some reduction in unit costs as more machines are sold. Manufacturers are looking at ways to reduce the cost of scanners by dispensing with gantry motion or by using fewer detectors.

There is presently interest in three-dimensional image acquisition which utilizes information throughout the axial field of view rather than in single planes. This may increase sensitivity four-fold where count rates are inherently low, as in [¹⁸F]dopa studies (Cherry et al., 1991). Thus three-dimensional image acquisition might be used to reduce scan times, enabling a greater throughput of patients.

Straightforward clinical studies can often use much simplified protocols, with static as opposed to dynamic acquisition. Where the brain is studied no measured attenuation correction need be performed, as a mathematical model for attenuation correction gives good results. These two factors reduce the time needed to perform PET imaging, allowing more patients to be scanned during a working day.

INDICATIONS FOR CLINICAL PET IMAGING

A variety of clinical applications for PET have recently emerged. The main areas where it is useful are cardiology, neurology and oncology.

PET in Cardiology

Ischaemic heart disease is the leading cause of death for men and women in the UK, accounting for 27% of all deaths (National Audit Office, 1989). Although there are many imaging techniques useful to cardiologists, imaging with ¹³NH₃ and ¹⁸FDG can accurately identify viable myocardium in patients with ischaemic disease (Marshall et al., 1983). The ¹³NH₃ uptake measures perfusion, while ¹⁸FDG measures glucose metabolism. If an area of absent or reduced perfusion appears to take up ¹⁸FDG, viability is probable. This variation in uptake between the two tracers is termed 'mismatch' (Figure 21.3). There is a high morbidity associated with revascularization, but if such patients survive the postoperative period significant gains in life expectancy are made. The high costs of PET imaging may be recouped if it can accurately identify patients who will benefit, given that a bypass graft operation costs over £4000 (National Audit Office, 1989).

In one study, 93 patients were followed up over 13 months, and mismatch of ¹³NH₃ versus ¹⁸FDG was found to predict patients likely to benefit from revascularization (Di Carli et al., 1994).

PET in Neurology

In the UK 40 000 people have epileptic seizures at least once per week, while over 50% of seizure sufferers have normal computed tomography

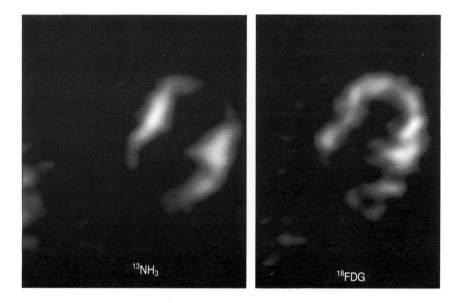

Figure 21.3   Mismatch of perfusion (^{13}NH$_3$, left) and glucose metabolism (^{18}FDG, right). This is seen at the top of each image corresponding to viable myocardium at the apex and anterior wall of the heart.

(CT) or magnetic resonance imaging (MRI) studies (Maisey and Jeffrey, 1991). PET has been shown to be helpful in localizing foci. Where surgery is considered, PET scanning may eliminate the need for depth electrode tests (Engel et al., 1990). Epileptic foci show up as decreased uptake of ^{18}FDG between seizures, but there may be increased uptake when these are taking place. An electroencephalogram (EEG) is performed during the uptake period following injection in order that the electrical activity in the regions under study is known.

Dementia is a prevalent problem among the elderly and will entail an enormous cost in an ageing population. There are characteristic uptake patterns of ^{18}FDG in dementia of Alzheimer's type (DAT) (Figure 21.4), making possible its differentiation from other types of dementia or depression as well as from Parkinsonism (Kumar, 1993).

Parkinsonism may also be investigated using [^{18}F]dopa, which demonstrates dopamine activity in the putamen and caudate nucleii of the brain. Recent advances in technology may permit its use as a clinical test, one application of which might be screening individuals with familial incidence of the disease (Eidelberg, 1992).

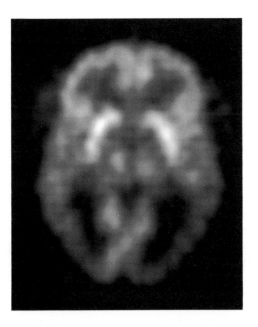

Figure 21.4   ¹⁸FDG brain scan of patient with Alzheimer's disease. Note bilateral reduction in tracer uptake, hence glucose metabolism, posteriorly.

PET in Oncology

Cancer cells metabolize glucose at a greater rate than normal tissue (Newsholme et al., 1985). Because uptake reflects glucose metabolism, PET with ¹⁸FDG is useful in:

1. Staging malignant disease, for example in carcinoma of the bronchus.
2. Differentiating benign from malignant disease, for example lung nodules.
3. Assessment of treatment of, for example, glioma.
4. Checking for disease recurrence as in, for example, lymphoma.
5. Survey in conditions such as malignant melanoma.

Breast cancer is the most common malignant disease in women, killing 13 000 annually (Central Office of Information, 1994). PET scanning with ¹⁸FDG is helpful in that it can identify axillary lymph node involvement non-invasively. This is a key prognosticator and may reduce the financial care burden by determination of optimal management (Institute for Clinical PET, Breast Cancer Team, 1994).

Another specific indication is the use of ¹⁸FDG to determine the nature of solitary lung nodules. Even with CT, up to 40% of nodules removed at surgery prove benign (Institute for Clinical PET, Solitary Pulmonary Nodule Team, 1994). Where attenuation-corrected PET images of the chest are acquired, a simple quantitative measure of ¹⁸FDG uptake known as the standardized uptake value (SUV) may be performed to assess whether a lesion is benign or malignant. This may, in turn, avoid thoracotomy.

It is possible to look for spread of a known malignancy or to seek the site of an unknown primary tumour by means of abutting several 10-cm depths of field in a whole-body PET scan (Figure 21.5). Data are collected for 5 minutes at each bed position; attenuation correction is not generally performed, but if a particular volume needs to be investigated this is studied separately in the same session.

Many tumours take up amino acids preferentially because of rapid cell division. [¹¹C]Methionine is particularly useful in the brain

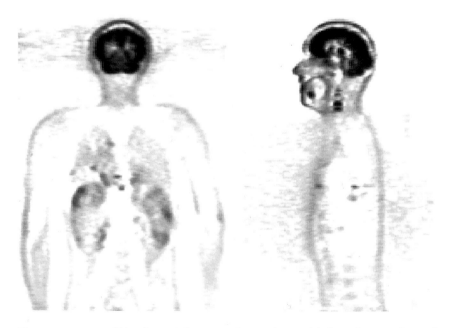

Figure 21.5   Half-body ¹⁸FDG scan of a patient with lymphoma. Several regions of increased uptake can be seen, suggesting active disease.

(Bergstrom et al., 1983). The tumour/background ratio with this tracer is higher, giving rise to greater certainty as to the extent of a lesion (Figure 21.6). It is generally used together with ¹⁸FDG sequentially in the same session to optimize PET study of a brain tumour.

One advantage of PET imaging in the brain is that it makes possible differentiation between necrotic or fibrosed areas and recurrence at the margins of a treated tumour (Di Chiro et al., 1988).

One factor which can limit the use of PET is that morphological information is not always good. Image registration of PET images with corresponding CT or magnetic resonance images is of help, as any areas of abnormal function seen on the PET image may be mapped on to the associated anatomical features. This is exacting to perform, requiring similar positioning for both studies and compatible computer systems. It then takes a skilled individual some time to align the scans ready for reporting. Alignment to within 3 mm is possible, which is well within the resolution of PET images (Hill et al., 1994). Automated registration systems have been reported (Mangin et al., 1994) and may make this a more practical everyday technique.

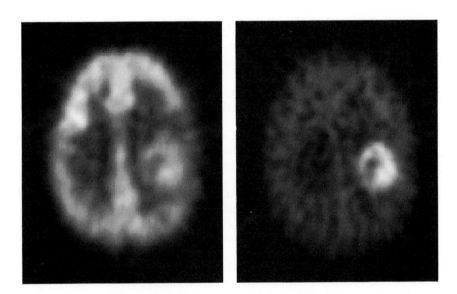

Figure 21.6   ¹⁸FDG (left) and [¹¹C]methionine (right) brain study. Note that the ¹⁸FDG image yields more morphological detail, but that the tumour stands out against its surroundings with the amino acid tracer.

SUMMARY

PET has been in existence for almost 20 years, and is now finding important uses as a clinical imaging modality. For certain groups of patients, such as those with cancer or heart disease, the technique has proven highly effective in diagnosis and management. PET can be used to select patients who are most likely to benefit from invasive procedures and thus to avoid such intervention for those unlikely to benefit. The other transaxial modalities of CT and MRI are an important adjunct in terms of the corresponding morphological information. PET may not become as widely used as conventional radionuclide imaging, but it is likely to have a valuable role to play as health care advances. Clinical PET imaging is likely to become more widespread as applications are proven and as the technology becomes both cheaper and simpler to use.

References

Bergstrom, M., Collins, V.P., Ehrin, E. et al. (1983) Discrepancies in brain tumour extent as shown by computed tomography and positron emission tomography using 68-Ga EDTA 11-C glucose and 11-C methionine *Journal of Computer Assisted Tomography* **7**: 1062–1066.

Central Office of Information (1994) *Britain – An Official Handbook*, London: HMSO.

Cherry, S.R., Dahlbom, M., Hoffman, E.J. (1991) Evaluation of a 3D reconstruction algorithm for multi-slice PET scanners. *Physical Medicine and Biology* **37**: 779–790.

Di Carli, M.F., Davidson, M., Little, R. et al. (1994) Value of metabolic imaging with positron emission tomography for evaluating prognosis in patients with coronary artery disease and left ventricular dysfunction. *American Journal of Cardiology* **73**: 527–533.

Di Chiro, G., Oldfield, E., Wright, D.C. et al. (1988) Cerebral necrosis after radiotherapy or intraarterial chemotherapy for brain tumours: PET and neuropathologic studies. *American Journal of Rontgenology* **150**: 189–197.

Eidelberg, D. (1992) Positron emission tomography studies in Parkinsonism. *Neurological Clinics* **10**: 421–433.

Engel, Jr, J., Henry, T.R., Risinger, M.W. et al. (1990) Presurgical evaluation for partial epilepsy: relative contributions of chronic depth electrode recordings versus FDG-PET and scalp sphenoidal ictal EEG. *Neurology* **40**: 1670–1677.

Hill, D., Edwards, P., Hawkes, D. (1994) Fusing medical images. *Image Processing* **6**: 22–25.

Institute for Clinical PET, Breast Cancer Team (1994) *Clinical Application and Economic Implications of PET in the Assessment of Axillary Lymph Node Involvement in Breast Cancer; A Retrospective Study.* Arlington: Institute for Clinical PET.

Institute for Clinical PET, Solitary Pulmonary Nodule Team (1994) *Clinical Application and Economic Implications of PET in the Assessment of Solitary Pulmonary Nodules; A Retrospective Study.* Arlington: Institute for Clinical PET.

Kumar, A. (1993) Functional brain imaging in late life depression and dementia. *Journal of Clinical Psychiatry* **54** (Suppl): 21–25.

Maisey, M., Jeffery, P. (1991) Clinical applications of positron emission tomography. *British Journal of Clinical Practice* **45**: 265–272.

Mangin, J.F., Frouin, V., Bloch, I. et al. (1994) Fast nonsupervised 3D registration of PET and MR images of the brain. *Journal of Cerebral Blood Flow and Metabolism* **14**: 749–762.

Marshall, R.L., Tillisch, J.H., Phelp, M.E. et al. (1983) Identification and differentiation of resting myocardial ischaemia and infarction in man with positron computed tomography ^{18}F labelled fluorodeoxyglucose and ^{13}N-ammonia. *Circulation* **67**: 766–778.

National Audit Office (1989) *NHS Coronary Heart Disease.* London: HMSO.

Newsholme, E.A., Crabtree, B., Ardawi, M.S. (1985) The role of high rates of glycolysis and glutamine in utilization in rapidly dividing cells. *Bioscience Reports* **5**: 393–400.

Spinks, T.J., Jones, T., Gilardi, M.C. et al. (1988) Physical performance of the latest generation of commercial positron scanner. *IEEE Transactions on Nuclear Science* **35**: 721–725.

22

The Future of Antibody Imaging, Research and Clinical Applications

Keith E. Britton and Maria Granowska

INTRODUCTION

The cancer cell differs from the normal cell in a number of subtle ways. This is because it possesses genes called *oncogenes* which have short sequences of DNA that differ from the normal sequence. The possession of such genetic differences leads to the disruption of the synthesis of suppressor proteins that control cell growth or the amplification of factors that stimulate cell growth, so that a cancer develops in an uncontrolled way and metastasizes to other tissues. As a result of these different biochemical processes, the cell surfaces of cancer cells differ in their properties from those of the normal cells. For example, the normal ovarian cell has a particular (HMFG) glycoprotein cover with many branching sugar chains over its surface. The equivalent ovarian cancer cell has a loss of many of these sugar chains so that the core protein of the HMFG glycoprotein is exposed. An antibody called SM3 made against a sequence of five amino acids that make up part of this exposed core protein reacts 17 times better with an ovarian cancer cell than with the normal ovarian cell. Such an antibody, if labelled with a radionuclide such as technetium-99m, is used to image ovarian cancer and distinguish it from normal ovarian tissue which only takes up very

The colour plate section for this article appears between p. 244 and p. 245.

little antibody (Granowska et al., 1993a). This is the basis of radio-immunoscintigraphy (RIS), the technique for imaging cancer (and other tissues) using a radiolabelled monoclonal antibody.

RIS differs from all radiological techniques since it is not using a physical property of the tumour such as size, shape, position, echogenicity, attenuation of X-rays, proton or water content, etc. It is using the essential cancerousness of the cell to distinguish it from the normal cell. It takes time for an antibody to be taken up by a tumour so the patient is imaged serially, usually at 10 minutes, 6 hours and 24 hours after the injection of the radiolabelled antibody. *Specific uptake* of the antibody by the tumour increases with time, whereas non-specific uptake, after the initial distribution, reduces with time as the blood is cleared of the antibody, for example in a vascular tumour such as a fibroid. The imaging is undertaken using a conventional gamma camera, which is available in every nuclear medicine department.

THE MONOCLONAL ANTIBODY

An antibody is a protein, a γ globulin, which the body produces in response to many foreign substances called *antigens*. The part of the antigen that stimulates lymphocytes to produce antibodies is called the *epitope* which may have components of sugar molecules and amino acids. Other chemicals can be antigenic if they are attached to larger molecules such as proteins. The normal way that the body reacts to, for example, a flu injection is to make a whole host of antibodies to different parts of the flu vaccine. This is called a polyclonal response. However, each particular lymphocyte only makes one particular antibody against one particular antigen. Clearly, for imaging it would be best to have one uniform antibody that reacted with a particular known antigen. Such an antibody is called a *monoclonal antibody* because the single lymphocyte that produces it is grown up as a family of lymphocytes, a clone.

Most monoclonal antibodies used clinically are prepared from mice. The mouse is immunized with the particular tumour extract or other tissue, its spleen is removed and the lymphocytes are then taken and fused with a mouse myeloma line. These hybrid lymphocytes are able to grow and divide and form a hybridoma. The hybrid lymphocytes are separated singly into little wells with culture medium. They are allowed to grow up, each clone producing one antibody. Each antibody is tested for its *specificity* to the chosen cancer or other tissue antigen and its *affinity*, i.e. its ability to bind tightly to that antigen.

Once a chosen monoclonal antibody has been selected that particular lymphocyte culture is increased in fermentation chambers so that a reasonable production of the monoclonal antibody is obtained. This is then purified and tested for stability, affinity and immunoreactivity with the chosen antigen. The Medical Control Agency requires that such production is undertaken in special laboratories meeting 'good manufacturing practice' standards. They require the application of extensive and expensive testing to make sure that the antibody is free of any remotely possible contamination, for example, from 14 mouse viruses which rarely affect man. It is the expense and time required to meet these regulatory requirements that make monoclonal antibodies difficult to obtain commercially.

The monoclonal antibody is a complexed molecule (Figure 22.1).

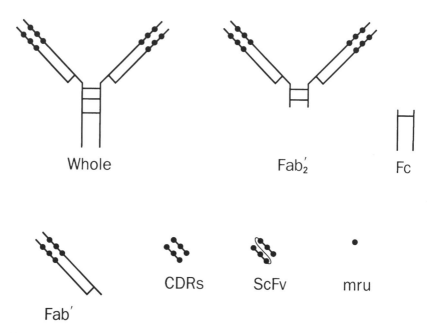

Figure 22.1   The whole antibody is represented by two heavy chains, two light chains outside the heavy chains and the Fc portion which is the tail of the heavy chains. Sulphur–sulphur bridges are shown linking the chains. The Fab$'_2$ antibody is obtained when the Fc portion, top right, is removed. Fab' is made up of a light and heavy chain joined together as in the whole antibody. Complementarity determinant regions (CDRs), three on each chain, are shown. A single chain fragment with the hypervariable region (ScFv) containing CDRs is created by genetic engineering. A molecular recognition unit (mru) is a single CDR.

Only a very small part of the whole structure reacts with the epitope of the antigen. These reactive parts are called *complementarity determinant regions* (CDRs) and are loops of 10–25 amino acids which are different in each antibody. They are specially arranged to interact together with the corresponding part of the epitope and held in position by a framework of supporting chains of amino acids. Two of these chains of amino acids are called *light chains* and two are called *heavy chains*. They connect together to form a hinge region which is connected to a tail called the *Fc portion*. This portion in some monoclonal antibodies can react with the cells of the liver, bone marrow and reticuloendothelial system non-specifically.

It is possible to divide the antibody into fragments by using proteolytic enzymes, thereby removing the Fc portion of the antibody. The biggest fragment contains all four chains and is called a *Fab'$_2$*. A smaller fragment contains only one heavy and one light chain and is called a *Fab fragment*. Even smaller fragments, called a *single chain Fv*, can be made; also single domain antibodies and even molecular recognition units consisting of just one or more CDRs can be made. These retain the specificity and selectivity of the antibody for the antigen but their ability to bind to the cancer cell becomes roughly progressively weaker the smaller the fragment. Much of the progress in monoclonal antibodies is in developing stable high-affinity fragments which, being small, have the advantage of deeper tumour penetration. This is a requirement for radioimmunotherapy (RIT). Fragments have a disadvantage of more rapid metabolism and rapid clearance from the blood, often by filtration and reabsorption in the proximal tubules of the kidneys where the radionuclide metal is deposited. For imaging, whole murine antibodies are satisfactory.

THE RADIONUCLIDE

Technetium-99m is the radionuclide of choice for nuclear medicine, because of its ready availability from a generator which is renewed each week, its low cost, and its short half-life of 6 hours. This allows a relatively large amount of activity (600 MBq) to be given, but with the rapid decay the total radiation dose to the patient is of the order of 4 mSv. This is well within the dose regarded as being of negligible risk by the International Commission on Radiation Protection and about equivalent to twice the annual radiation background received in London and one-fifth that received in Cornwall or Aberdeen. Recording a radiograph of the kidneys would give about the same effective dose.

The importance of the signal in imaging cannot be overstressed. The higher the count rate, the better the signal, the less the noise (which is based on the square root of the signal count), the earlier and the smaller is the tumour identified. For some time it was not possible to label monoclonal antibodies with technetium-99m in a stable way, but this was resolved by the reduction technique of Schwarz. In this the cysteine links through sulphur bridges at the hinge region of the antibody are reduced by 2-mecaptoethanol. Then a bone-scanning kit provides tin to reduce technetium-99m, enabling stable linkage of technetium-99m to the antibody through bonding across four sulphur bridges. This original technique has been modified (Mather and Ellison, 1990) and is now in routine use for a number of monoclonal antibodies. Newer methods of technetium-99m labelling involve either attaching a linker to the antibody which can then bind the technetium-99m, or prelabelling the linker with technetium-99m and attaching it to the antibody. These later methods are particularly required when using fragments for imaging.

Indium-111 has a half-life of 67 hours and has to be purchased at considerable expense on each occasion. Its longer half-life means a lower amount can be given, and a typical administered dose is 120 MBq, giving a radiation effective dose of 24 mSv. It is clearly less advantageous for imaging than is technetium-99m. It used to be thought that it took a long time for the antibody to bind to the tumour, but in fact over 75% of a typical whole murine monoclonal antibody is bound to tumour within 12 hours; thus imaging may be completed within 24 hours using the technetium-99m radiolabel. A typical blood clearance rate ($t_{1/2}$) of a technetium-99m or indium-111 labelled whole monoclonal antibody is 24 hours. It is important to check that the radiolabelling of the monoclonal antibody does not alter its immunoreactivity adversely.

It is essential that the gamma camera is optimized for the particular radionuclide and that it has daily quality control so that its performance is at its best to enable small recurrences to be identified. The gamma camera is set with a general-purpose low-energy parallel collimator and set up for technetium-99m with a peak of 140 keV and a window of 20%. Alternatively, for monoclonal antibodies labelled with indium-111, a medium energy parallel hole collimator is used and peaking is done for the two energies of indium-111 (171 and 274 keV with 20% windows). Single photon emission tomography (SPET), where the gamma camera is rotated around the patient, is used to improve the imaging of the pelvis and the paraaortic region and liver when undertaking RIS in colorectal, prostate and gynaecological tumours.

CLINICAL APPLICATIONS

RIS is designed to answer important clinical questions in the diagnosis and management of patients with cancer that cannot be answered by conventional and advanced radiological techniques.

It is used to demonstrate subclinical and subradiological disease. For example: 1-mm thin plaques of ovarian cancer spread over the peritoneum; the involved lymph node that is less than 1 cm in diameter; and the recurrence of colorectal or prostatic cancer in the pelvis.

RIS can demonstrate primary and recurrent cancer before there is an elevation of serum markers. For example, a Dukes' C staged colorectal cancer, that is when the primary tumour has associated with it involved nodes at the time of surgery, has a 50% chance of recurrence within 1 year. RIS is able to demonstrate such recurrence before there is a rise in the serum carcinoembryonic antigen (CEA) because the tumour has to be of a certain size to liberate sufficient markers to increase the level of the marker in the plasma over that which is metabolized in the liver and over the normal variation of the plasma level.

If serum markers are elevated, RIS can be used to localize the site of the disease, often by using a radiolabelled version of the monoclonal antibody against the particular serum marker.

After treatment of cancer there is often a radiologically identifiable mass, but neither computed tomography (CT), magnetic resonance imaging (MRI) nor ultrasound can distinguish whether such a mass contains viable tumour or is just fibrosis or infection. The specificity of the monoclonal antibody is such that, provided serial imaging is done, specific uptake by a tumour can be distinguished from the other causes of the mass.

A 'second-look' operation is often done to determine whether therapy has been successful. RIS can identify tumour recurrences or demonstrate that chemotherapy has been successful if imaging is done before and after the therapy.

The potential contribution of RIS to cancer management is thus considerable.

PATIENT PROTOCOL

A detailed explanation of the test to the patient, and to medical and nursing colleagues is essential. Informed signed consent is advisable, since most RIS studies are undertaken under ethics committee control.

No skin test is advised, as this may sensitize the patient to produce human antibodies against the murine antibodies (human antimouse antibodies (HAMA)). Patients with a history of allergy to foreign protein or with a severe atopic predisposition should not be injected with monoclonal antibody.

The patient receives typically 600 MBq with 0.5 mg of the chosen monoclonal antibody labelled with technetium-99m and is then positioned supine on the imaging couch. For abdominal cancers the camera is positioned over the pelvis first and 800 000 counts are collected per view for a set of two anterior and two posterior images and a squat view of the pelvis. Images are typically obtained at 10 minutes, 6 hours and 22 hours, with SPET at 6 and 22 hours. When indium-111 is used, images are taken at 10 minutes, 22 hours and at 48–72 hours.

IMAGE INTERPRETATION

The 10-minute image shows no specific uptake of the antibody. Therefore, it is the template with which the later images can be compared. Remembering that specific uptake increases with time, whereas after the initial distribution non-specific uptake decreases with time during the first 24 hours, it will be evident that if something is seen on the 6- and, even more significantly, on the 22-hour images that was not present on the 10-minute image it is likely to represent tumour uptake. Some urinary activity and bowel activity may appear at later times. It is always important to have the patient empty their bladder before each image and empty their bowel before the next morning's image. Typically, vascular tumours which are not cancer will show high uptake on the 10-minute image and that uptake will decrease with time as the blood-pool activity decreases. A cyst will show as a defect in the image unchanged all the way through, unless it is a malignant cyst when uptake will be seen in the wall of the cavity increasing with time.

The liver can have a variety of changes. A large tumour will show on the 10-minute image as a defect with very little change between the next two images. A slightly smaller tumour will show as a defect on the first image and then have increasing uptake as a halo around it on the later images. A smaller tumour still will have a defect on the 10-minute image and will then disappear into the normal liver tissue on the later images, since its uptake is equivalent to the normal tissue. Lastly, a very small metastasis may show no abnormality on the early images but appear as a focal area of increased uptake (more than the normal liver uptake) on the 22-hour image.

By using technetium-99m as the radiolabel, RIS is as good as CT and ultrasound in picking up liver metastases of colorectal cancer (Granowska et al., 1993b). This is not true for indium-111 labelled monoclonal antibodies, since the metabolism of the antibody by the reticuloendothelial system deposits indium-111 in the liver where it may obscure the subtle changes outlined above. Indium-111 is also deposited to some extent in the gut, marrow and other reticuloendothelial systems with time, so it may be less easy to distinguish a tumour recurrence from normal tissue background activity.

Clinical examples of technetium-99m and indium-111 labelled antibodies in ovarian cancer, colorectal cancer and ocular melanoma are shown in Figures 22.2, 22.3 and Plates 4–6.

IMAGE ANALYSIS

Since specific uptake of the monoclonal antibody increases with time, the easiest analysis is to subtract the earliest image (taken at 10 minutes) from the latest image (at 22 hours). The differences between the two images will enhance tumour sites. In order to undertake this reliably, the two images must be superimposed perfectly. For this, prior

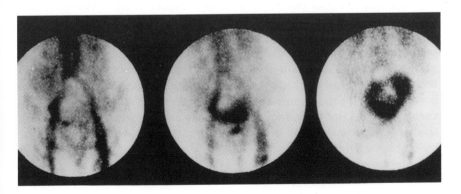

Figure 22.2 Ovarian cancer (technetium-99m SM3 (IRCF)). Anterior views of the pelvis at 10 minutes (left), 6 hours (centre) and 24 hours (right). Increasing uptake with time of the technetium-99m SM3 in the tumour is seen. There is a central defect due to necrosis. (Courtesy of *International Journal of Biological Markers* (1990) **5**: 89–96.)

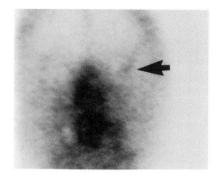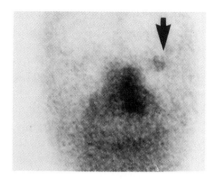

Figure 22.3   Ocular melanoma (technetium-99m Fab 225.28S (Sorin)). Anterior views of the face at 6 hours. (Left) A normal patient; (right) uptake in an ocular melanoma in the right eye (arrow).

images of markers labelled with cobalt-57 or barium-133 for technetium-99m or indium-111 imaging, respectively, are set on indelible marks made on the skin over prominent bony landmarks such as the symphysis pubis, anterior iliac crests, lower rib margins and xiphisternum. The marker images are recorded on the oscilloscope and transparent film is used to mark the relative positions of the points. When the patient comes back the radioactive markers are repositioned on the skin marks and the patient is moved until the markers superimpose on the transparent film obtained from the earlier image. The data are recorded by the computer system and a special translation rotation program is used to superimpose the markers from the late image more precisely onto the early image. Then the program takes the actual patient image at 22 hours and moves it through the same pattern as the marker images so that the late and the early images are superimposed. Image subtraction is performed after scaling each image such that all images have the same total count content. The disadvantage of this approach is that there may be a tendency to over- or under-subtract the early image from late image.

A more sophisticated approach is called *kinetic analysis with probability mapping*. A change-detection algorithm is used to compare the two images. If there has been no change between the two images when they are compared then a line of identity is created. If there are differences between the two images that are significant, these will be seen as deviations from the line of identity representing no change. These deviations from the line of identity can be tested using a χ^2 statistic and the significance of the deviation from the line of identity can be determined

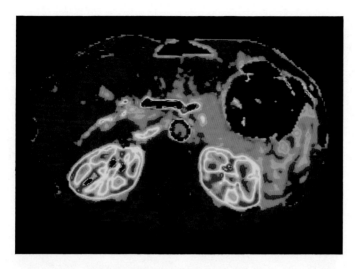

Plate 1 Perfusion image of the upper abdomen. The combination of high resolution and quantifiable perfusion information is demonstrated by the clear distinction of perfusion values within the renal cortex and medulla and the splenic pathways. Colour scale: black – 0 ml min⁻¹ml⁻¹; blue – 1.5 ml min⁻¹ml⁻¹; pink – 5 ml min⁻¹ml⁻¹.

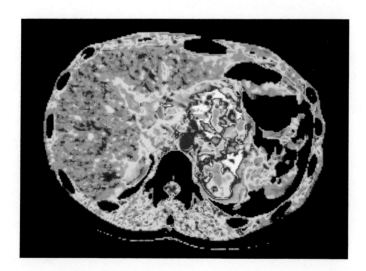

Plate 2 Functional image demonstrating proportional arterial blood flow. A low proportion of arterial perfusion is seen within the liver, reflecting the dominance of the portal system in perfusing the normal liver. Structures outside the liver show predominantly arterial perfusion. Colour scale: black – no arterial; blue – 25% arterial; pink/white – 100% arterial.

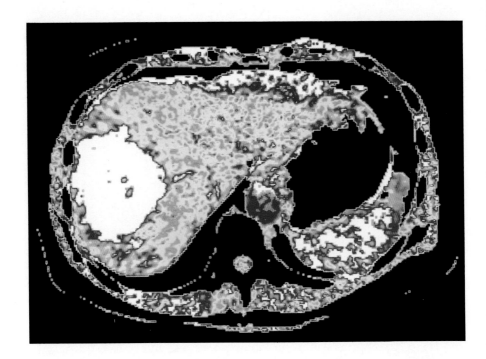

Plate 3 Functional image, demonstrating proportional arterial perfusion in a liver containing a large metastasis. Total arterial perfusion in the metastasis is indicated by its white colour, the colour of the remainder of the liver indicates approximately 50% perfusion, i.e. higher than in a normal liver. This increase is often seen where hepatic metastases are present, even in areas of the liver which are unaffected. Colour scale: as in Plate 2.

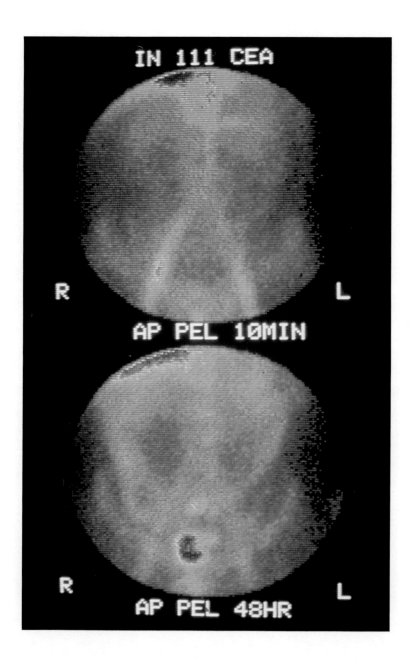

Plate 4 Colorectal cancer (indium-111 anti-CEA (C 46)). Anterior views of the abdomen and pelvis at 10 minutes (top) and 48 hours (bottom). Increased uptake in the pelvis is seen in red in the later image due to tumour uptake.

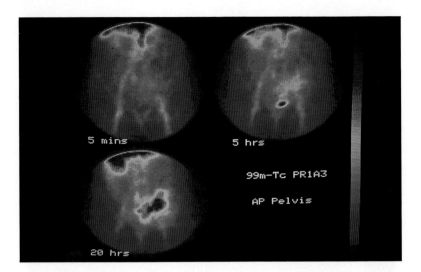

Plate 5 Colorectal cancer (technetium-99m PR1A3 (ICRF)). Anterior views of the abdomen at 5 minutes (top left), 5 hours (top right) and 20 hours (bottom). Increasing uptake in the left iliac fossa (in red) is seen in the recurrence of colorectal cancer at 20 hours.

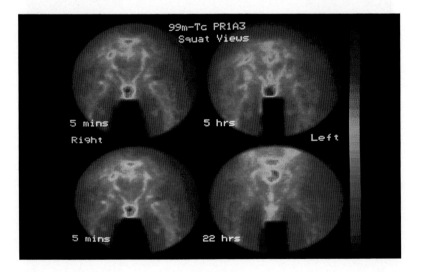

Plate 6 Colorectal cancer (technetium-99m PR1A3 (ICRF)). Squat views of the pelvis at 5 minutes (top and bottom left), 5 hours (top right) and 22 hours (bottom right). Decreasing vascularity with time is seen in the genitalia anteriorly with time. Clearance of non-specific activity is seen in red. Increasing uptake with time is seen posteriorly in the rectal cancer (in red).
(Courtesy of *European Journal of Nuclear Medicine* (1993) **20:** 690–698.)

as a probability value. The probability values are then plotted as colours at the sites of the deviations, for example $P < 0.001$ in red, $P < 0.01$ in yellow, and $P < 0.05$ in blue. In this way a new image is produced, called a *probability map*, where only the significant changes between the two conventional images are recorded. From this map very small tumours can be identified, for example recurrences of ovarian cancer of less than half a centimetre (Granowska et al., 1988) and axillary node involvement in breast cancer.

NEW TWO- AND THREE-STAGE IMAGING

The merits of imaging with radiolabelled antibodies have often been ignored by commercial companies as they seek to use the same technique to target radionuclide-therapy labelled antibodies to treat cancer. This is much more difficult, due to three main reasons. Firstly, in imaging it does not matter if only the outer shell of the tumour takes up the antibody (the signal from the tumour will be evident) but for therapy the antibody with its therapy label must target the middle of the tumour. Secondly, the amount of antibody and its residence time on the tumour can be quite small for imaging, whereas for therapy it must bring a reasonable amount of the radiotherapy radionuclide to irradiate the tumour over a prolonged period. Thirdly, and most importantly, for imaging it does not matter that the normal tissues are bathed in radiolabelled antibody since the radiation dose is very small, whereas for therapy the irradiation of normal tissues by radiotherapy radionuclide-labelled antibody not taken up by tumour (about 97% of the administered antibody) is potentially harmful to the bone marrow and gives a poor therapeutic ratio. In order to overcome this problem, a series of clever strategies has been devised involving two or three stages of targeting the tumour. The most widely tested is the *avidin–biotin* system (Paganelli et al., 1993).

Biotin is a small molecule (vitamin B_6) which binds very strongly to the protein avidin at four different sites. Biotin is attached to the monoclonal antibody chosen to bind to the cancer and this non-radioactive combination is injected first. Avidin is injected 2 or 3 days later after the antibody has been metabolized in the blood and normal tissues, but not that on the tumour. Avidin therefore binds to the biotin attached to the antibody attached to the tumour. Non-bound avidin clears any unbound biotin-linked antibody into the liver and reticuloendothelial system. One day later radiolabelled biotin is injected. For imaging, the radiolabel may be indium-111 or technetium-99m; for therapy it may be yttrium-90. The third stage with the biotin-linked radionuclide targets the avidin which is bound to the biotin to the antibody to the tumour. Unbound biotin-linked radiotherapy radionuclide clears rapidly through the kidneys so the irradiation of normal tissues is short, whereas the residence time of the radiolabelled biotin attached to the tumour is long, giving a good therapeutic ratio. Variations on this theme for imaging include indium-111 labelled avidin with biotin-linked antibody injected first; or technetium-99m labelled biotin with avidinated antibody injected first.

An alternative approach is to use a bifunctional antibody. These can be created by linking two Fab or Fv groups together, one group binding to the cancer and the other to a radiotherapy labelled molecule called a ligand. The linkage between the two fragments may be chemical or through genetic engineering. The bifunctional antibody (non-radioactive) is injected first and binds the tumour. Unbound bifunctional antibody is cleared into the liver and reticuloendothelial system. Two or three days later the radiolabelled ligand is injected and picks out the bifunctional antibody bound to tumour. Unbound radiolabelled ligand is excreted rapidly through the kidneys, again giving a good therapeutic ratio (Britton et al., 1991).

A further variant on this approach is to use an oligonucleotide, which is a small molecule made up of base pairs in the same way that DNA is made up. As DNA has the ability to replicate it has 'sense' and 'antisense' complementary chains. For the two-step approach a sense oligonucleotide is attached to the monoclonal antibody designed to target the cancer. The radiolabel is attached to an antisense oligonucleotide which will only bind with the sense oligonucleotide attached to the tumour, thereby targeting the radiolabel for imaging or therapy. These developments in the field are tested out by using imaging radionuclides, but are designed for radioimmunotherapy.

GENETIC ENGINEERING

The formation of all proteins by cells is controlled by genes, and antibodies are no exception. It is possible to isolate the genes that produce the heavy chains and the genes that produce the light chains and combine them in a yeast or in a bacterial form called a 'plasmid'. The plasmid will then produce the chosen antibody as well as its own proteins from its genetic intruder and its own genes. This is similar to the way that a virus infects the cell and injects its own DNA or RNA into the host genetic DNA or RNA and, therefore, replicates itself and its own instructions to build itself again. In fact, bacteriophages can be used to aid this genetic transformation of the host plasmid. This ability to transfer human fragments of genes has been helped by the development of the polymerase chain reaction (PCR), which is a method of replicating DNA or RNA sequences millions of times over through using a particular enzyme polymerase.

This genetic material in plasmids may be combined together in random fashion to make libraries of heavy- and light-chain synthesizing systems. In this way it is hoped that new monoclonal antibody-like molecules will be developed with quite different binding properties than can be found in nature. Moreover, by using human material the human antimouse response can be avoided. The HAMA response is not a problem for imaging, but is a problem when large amounts of mouse monoclonal antibody are used in therapy.

At present, there are available chimeric antibodies where the Fc portion of the mouse antibody is replaced by a human Fc, and human reshaped antibodies (also called 'CDR grafted antibodies') where both the Fc portion and the framework of the mouse antibody are replaced by human antibody, leaving only the CDRs to be of murine origin. There are further advantages for genetically engineered molecules. For example, a sequence that will bind technetium-99m can be introduced into the peptide, or else the binding affinity may be enhanced by changing one amino acid for another. In this way quite novel peptides can be produced which are based on, but no longer are, monoclonal antibodies. They have more in common with receptor binding peptides such as [^{111}In]octreotide which is also used for imaging cancer. Indeed, there is a convergence between the receptor peptides that are being developed and synthesized and the monoclonal antibody derived genetically engineered peptide molecules that are being created. All are examples of the *binder–bindee concept*, where a bindee is chosen for radiolabelling and to react with a specific binder property on the tumour cell surface.

The field is progressing further with the use of oligonucleotides themselves as imaging and therapy agents. In this case they are made resistant to destructive enzymes in the plasma. They can enter the cell and the cell nucleus. If the correct antisense sequence is chosen, they could bind directly with the particular abnormal oncogene sequence present in the cancer cell. The potential for imaging and therapy in these ways is enormous.

CONCLUSION

RIS is a robust imaging technique whose time has come. Its main use is the identification of cancer that cannot be detected clinically, radiologically or by serum markers. It also has uses in the identification of heart attacks (Manspeaker et al., 1993), deep vein thrombosis (Schaible and Alavi, 1991), and imaging infection through antibodies to white cells (Peltier et al., 1993), but its main use is in cancer. Developments of monoclonal antibodies for imaging and therapy of virtually every type of cancer are being researched in academic departments. Their applications are mainly limited not by science but by the hostile regulatory environment that prevents their rapid and cost-effective commercial development.

References

Britton, K.E., Mather, S.J., Granowska, M. (1991) Radiolabelled monoclonal antibodies in oncology. III Radioimmunotherapy. *Nuclear Medicine Communications* **12:** 333–347.
Granowska, M., Nimmon, C.C., Britton, K.E. et al. (1988) Kinetic analysis and probability mapping applied to the detection of ovarian cancer by radioimmunoscintigraphy. *Journal of Nuclear Medicine* **29:** 599–607.
Granowska, M., Britton, K.E., Mather, S.J. et al. (1993a) Radioimmunoscintigraphy with technetium-99m labelled monoclonal antibody, SM3, in gynaecological cancer. *European Journal of Nuclear Medicine* **20:** 483–489.
Granowska, M., Britton, K.E., Mather, S.J. et al. (1993b) Radioimmunoscintigraphy with technetium-99m labelled monoclonal antibody, 1A3, in colorectal cancer. *European Journal of Nuclear Medicine* **20:** 690–698.
Manspeaker, P., Weisman, H.F., Schaible, T.F. (1993) Cardiovascular applications: current status of radioimmunoscintigraphy in the detection of myocardial necrosis using antimyosin, and deep vein thrombosis using antifibrin. *Seminars in Nuclear Medicine* **23:** 133–147.
Mather, S.J., Ellison, D. (1990) Reduction medicated technetium-99m labelling of monoclonal antibodies. *Journal of Nuclear Medicine* **31:** 692–697.
Paganelli, G., Malcovati, M., Fazio, F. (1993) Monoclonal antibody pretargetting techniques for tumour localisation; the avidin biotin system. *Nuclear Medicine Communications* **12:** 211–234.
Peltier, P., Potel, G., Lovat, E. et al. (1993) Detection of lung and bone infection with anti-granulocyte monoclonal antibody BW250/183 radiolabelled with $^{99}Tc^m$. *Nuclear Medicine Communications* **14:** 766–774.
Schaible, T.F., Alavi, A. (1991) Antifibrin scintigraphy in the diagnostic evaluation of acute deep venous thrombosis. *Seminars in Nuclear Medicine* **21:** 313–324.

23

Conformal Radiotherapy

Lynne Sterry

INTRODUCTION

Conformal therapy is a technique in which the spatial distribution of a high radiation dose is tailored to conform closely to the size and shape of the target volume in all three dimensions. In its simplest form, static conformal therapy utilizes shielding blocks placed in the path of a stationary beam to achieve field shaping. Modern treatment machines operating under computer control have made possible the more complex technique of dynamic conformal therapy. This is achieved by continuous variation of certain treatment parameters, for example, gantry rotation, during the exposure and, in its most advanced form, includes beam intensity modulation.

Whichever method is chosen, the objectives of conformal therapy are two-fold and interlinked. Firstly, the maximal exclusion of normal tissue from the beam should reduce the incidence of acute adverse reactions and chronic morbidity. As a consequence, this may lead to an improvement in the patient's quality of life even if the prognosis is unaffected. Secondly, as the tolerance of healthy tissues is inversely proportional to the volume irradiated, restriction of radiation to the tumour alone should facilitate dose escalation. It is postulated that increasing the radiation dose may result in improved local control for a number of tumour sites. The combined outcome of these two objectives should, therefore, be an improved therapeutic ratio.

The theoretical advantages of conformal therapeutic techniques have been discussed in the literature since the early 1900s. However, it was impossible to predetermine the dose distributions arising from these techniques with conventional two-dimensional planning methods, and the treatment was difficult to implement with the equipment available at the time. The concept of conformal therapy is therefore not new, but the resurgence of interest in recent years is largely a result of the rapid advances which have taken place in tumour imaging, computer planning software, treatment unit design and treatment verification. These developments have revolutionized the possibilities for conformal therapy in terms of the extent to which its objectives can be realized and the precision with which the techniques can be performed.

The planning and delivery of conformal radiotherapy involves many links in a chain, and for the chain to remain intact each of its links must receive the same attention in terms of research and development. Two potential weaknesses lie in the initial delineation of the *Clinical Target Volume* (ICRU, 1992) and the lack of reproducibility of the patient's position.

TUMOUR LOCALIZATION

The accuracy of the initial tumour-localization procedure is critical if treatment margins are to be reduced and excessive irradiation of normal tissues avoided. An important question to be answered before embarking on conformal treatment techniques is, therefore, whether the existing methods of localization are sufficiently precise to allow 'safety margins' of only a few millimetres; a geographical miss may contribute to failure to control the primary tumour and increase the risk of recurrence at the treatment margins. Despite rapid advances, all the currently available imaging modalities have their limitations and none can compete with the accuracy of histological assessment in determining the accurate extent of the primary tumour. As the delineation of the tumour can only be as accurate as the method used to visualize it, this stage of the treatment-planning process can probably be regarded as the weakest link in the chain, due to the uncertainties which surround it.

The ability of computed tomography (CT) scanning to visualize the volume to be treated throughout its entire length established the possibility of planning radiotherapy in all three dimensions. Manual outlining of the target on consecutive 'slices' is, however, time consuming and requires the clinician and/or dosimetrist to have a good knowledge of cross-sectional anatomy. The accuracy of the procedure is also dependent on the skill and patience of the operator and, where structure boundaries are not readily apparent, the process may not be reproducible. Although most planning systems provide an automatic contouring facility, this may only be useful for delineating the patient contour (i.e. the skin surface) and gross inhomogeneities such as lung tissue, as it is dependent on the recognition of density differences which may not exist between tumour and soft tissues. Delineation of the presumed target volume is therefore subjective, and the temptation to err on the side of caution may lead to the incorporation of wide margins, which negates the objective of minimizing normal-tissue irradiation. There is clearly a need for improvement in this stage of the planning process and in recognition of this, a number of workers are involved in the development of autocontouring methods and artificial-intelligence approaches using knowledge-based systems (Orhun et al., 1993).

PATIENT POSITIONING

The positioning of the patient to ensure the reproducibility of the daily irradiation geometry is a critical requirement in the planning and delivery of radiotherapy. The adoption of smaller treatment volumes for conformal therapy and the potential use of higher dose levels call for even greater precision if the tumour is to be fully encompassed and normal tissue tolerances not exceeded. The daily reproducibility of the patient's position must therefore be assured; one approach is to ensure secure immobilization and a number of studies have shown that the use of customized immobilization devices significantly reduces errors in patient positioning (Soffen et al., 1991; Rosenthal et al., 1993). The need to manufacture such devices individually inevitably adds to the pretreatment preparation in terms of time, staff involvement and costs, but their use may reduce patient set-up time, which is usually the most laborious part of the actual treatment procedure.

Portal films have been the conventional means of verifying the accuracy of the set-up on the treatment unit, but the efficacy of this method is limited, particularly for conformal therapy. Much attention has thus been devoted to the development of 'megavoltage' imaging (MVI). Such systems provide images of a quality comparable to, if not better than, those obtained by film and have the added advantage of rapid availability. Their digital format means they may readily be subject to on-line image processing and comparison with digitized simulator images or digitally reconstructed radiographs (DRRs) obtained from a set of CT scans.

At present, the majority of MVI systems produce two-dimensional images and enable comparison only of the position of bony landmarks within the patient; they do not illustrate the position of the actual tumour which is, of course, the real area of interest. Most devices can be used at all treatment angles, as they are attached to the linear accelerator gantry. However, the interpretation of anatomical structures is difficult on oblique views and may be even more confusing if non-coplanar fields are used. The presence of a beam-modifying device, such as a wedge filter, in the path of the beam tends to degrade the quality of the image, so it is possible that the choice of beam arrangement will be dictated by the need to produce a recognizable image rather than that which is optimum for treating the tumour or sparing normal tissues. In addition, the use of such verification systems may increase the treatment set-up time as the physical bulk of the imaging device may restrict the radiographer's access to the patient or, if the device is demountable, necessitate its repeated removal and reattachment. The total time for which the patient has to remain still on the treatment couch may therefore be increased, particularly if multiple fields need to be verified and, given that the majority of radiotherapy patients are elderly, the prolonged discomfort may actually increase the likelihood of movement.

The ability of on-line verification systems to quantify discrepancies between the patient's intended (simulated) position and his or her actual position on the treatment couch offers the potential to instigate remedial action before the commencement of the treatment exposure. This raises the question as to *who* decides if the set-up is sufficiently acceptable to proceed – the clinician, the radiographer or the computer?

CLINICAL BENEFIT

Smith (1990) states that, in order to justify the expense of adopting new technologies, there should be a demonstrable gain in quality of patient care, efficiency or safety. However, little work has been done to evaluate the *clinical* benefit that conformal therapy may offer in comparison with existing conventional methods of radiation treatment, although an ongoing prospective, randomized trial at the Royal Marsden Hospital is aiming to provide some of the answers (Tait et al., 1993).

Although it may be demonstrated graphically that treatment plans using multiple, non-coplanar, intricately shaped beams can reduce the volume of normal tissue irradiated, this may be of little consequence to the patient, as few, if any, normal tissues exceed their tolerance dose to appreciable volumes in the conventional treatment plan. Reduced normal-tissue exposure may also be at the expense of an increased risk of recurrence at the treatment margins, as the inherent limitations of existing imaging techniques means that microscopic invasion cannot be determined accurately. The small treatment margins used in conformal therapy make its precise delivery highly dependent on patient and organ immobility and the complexity of the set-up may increase the likelihood of human error. Conformal radiotherapy may thus be self-defeating in that local control rates could worsen.

Attempts to increase the tumour dose may result in a greater risk of acute and chronic toxicity, which will reduce the patient's quality of life; treatment-related morbidity may thus exceed any benefit gained from dose escalation in some tumour sites. The role of conformal therapy therefore needs to be defined carefully, so that it may be used to advantage in those patients who are potentially able to benefit from it; it would be a waste of resources to dedicate complex conformal technology to the treatment of, for example, those patients whose fate is determined by biological, rather than technological variables.

The introduction of any major new treatment technique should include a cost–benefit analysis in addition to clinical considerations. Conformal radiotherapy places considerable additional demands upon clinicians, physicists, mould-room technicians and radiographers in terms of both time and effort, and it may not make financial sense to provide a treatment that will offer only a marginal improvement in life for a few patients if a large percentage of the departmental budget is taken up and patient throughput decreased as a result of its implementation. The issue of cost has important implications for staffing levels and equipment in radiotherapy, and it is possible that many clinical departments could not afford to adopt conformal techniques, even if they wished to. According to a report from the Royal College of Radiologists (1991), the speciality is facing a manpower shortage that is threatening the standard of cancer treatment in this country. Provision of clinical oncologists has failed to keep up with the rising demand for cancer treatment, and therapeutic radiographers and medical physicists are also in short supply in certain parts of the country. In contrast, the standard of equipment available in the UK's radiotherapy centres is reported as being generally good. The Department of Health's interest in boosting the provision of linear accelerators may be due to the belief that patient throughput can be increased due to the short treatment times. However, it is the patient set-up, rather than the radiation exposure, which accounts for most of the treatment time and the increased complexity introduced by conformal techniques, onset field verification, etc., is likely to increase rather than decrease this time, and may even reduce the number of patients it is possible to treat in the working day.

Lichter (1991) states that conformal radiotherapy:

> *Is a testable hypothesis and one that should be allowed to succeed or fail based on the result of clinical trials, not on the result of theoretical speculation. Three-dimensional treatment planning and conformal dose delivery should be given the opportunity to show whether better outcomes can be produced compared to conventionally available treatment delivery techniques.*

It should, of course, be ensured that new conformal techniques are being compared to the highest standard of existing treatments; it is possible that if all institutions adopted the best current practice of conventional radiotherapy, the overall gains might outweigh any increments achievable by the use of conformal techniques at a few specialized centres. However, it is also possible that some patients may not be prepared to accept a 'low-tech' treatment if they know that state-of-the-art technology is available.

CONCLUSION

The potential clinical advantages of conformal therapy can only be evaluated by the use of prospective, randomized trials and not by comparison with historical controls. Researchers in the field of conformal therapy need first clearly to define the end-points for evaluation. Is the aim, for example, to increase survival rates, improve local control, or reduce morbidity, or all of these? Local control rates and normal-tissue complications resulting from conventional treatments need to be reviewed to provide an agreed baseline for evaluation. Only after completion of these studies could a direct comparison between conformal and standard treatment techniques be contemplated and the magnitude of any improvement quantified. A series of dose-escalation studies would then allow identification of the optimum dose level and treatment technique, as well as providing a preliminary indication of its effectiveness (Lichter, 1991). To ensure the most efficient use of limited health resources in the UK, it may be wise for one centre to co-ordinate such research to ensure the standardization and quality assurance of treatment protocols.

In conclusion, the implementation of conformal treatment techniques is likely to have a significant impact on the working practices of radiotherapy departments, but whether the effects are clinically beneficial or economically desirable is yet to be proven. Nevertheless, some of the innovations which have contributed to the development of three-dimensional therapy will no doubt be of value in improving the precision of radiation treatments in general.

References

International Commission on Radiation Units and Measurements (1992) *Prescribing, Recording and Reporting Photon Beam Therapy (ICRU 50)*. Bethesda, MD: ICRU.

Lichter, A.S. (1991) Three dimensional conformal radiation therapy: a testable hypothesis. *International Journal of Radiation Oncology, Biology, Physics* **21:** 853–855.

Orhun, U., Viggars, D.A., Shalev, S. (1993) Knowledge-based auto-contouring on CT image slices: application to carcinoma of the prostate. In: Minet, P. (ed) *Three-dimensional Treatment Planning. European Association of Radiology 5th Workshop*, Geneva, pp 27–32. Liége: World Health Organization.

Rosenthal, S.A., Roach, M., Goldsmith, B.J. et al. (1993) Immobilization improves the reproducibility of patient positioning during six-field conformal radiation therapy for prostate carcinoma. *International Journal of Radiation Oncology, Biology, Physics* **27:** 921–926.

Royal College of Radiologists (1991) *Medical Manpower and Workload in Clinical Oncology in the UK*. London: Board of the Faculty of Clinical Oncology, Royal College of Radiologists.

Smith, A.R. (1990) Evaluation of new radiation oncology technology. *International Journal of Radiation Oncology, Biology, Physics* **18:** 701–703.

Soffen, E.M., Hanks, G.E., Hwang, C.C. et al. (1991) Conformal static field therapy for low volume low grade prostate cancer with rigid immobilisation. *International Journal of Radiation Oncology, Biology, Physics* **20:** 141–146.

Tait, D.M., Nahum, A.E., Rigby, L. et al. (1993) Conformal radiotherapy of the pelvis: assessment of acute toxicity. *Radiotherapy and Oncology* **29:** 117–126.

24

Continuous Hyperfractionated Accelerated Radiotherapy

Cathy Williams

INTRODUCTION

Fractionation

It was in France during the 1920s that the fractionation of radiotherapy was first explained (Hall, 1978). It was noted previously, in experiments concerning the dose required to sterilize the testes of goats, that the skin reaction was reduced by dividing the treatment into a number of fractions. This reduction in the normal tissue reaction is one of the reasons why the majority of radiotherapy treatment courses given today are split into fractions.

Hyperfractionation

The choice of size of fractions can be described using the graph in Figure 24.1. Early-responding tissues are those which react during or shortly after a course of radiation treatment. Late-responding tissues are those which show a radiation response months after the completion of radiotherapy.

It should be noted that tumours generally behave as early-responding tissues, such as the skin and mucosa, where the surviving fraction of cells is only slightly reduced by increasing the dose per fraction. Vascular and connective tissue, which are late-responding, are greatly

CHART   257

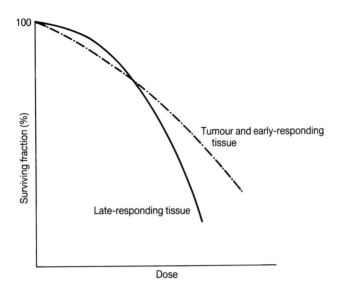

Figure 24.1   The increase in dose per fraction has less effect on the surviving fraction of cells in a tumour or early-responding tissues than on late-responding tissues.

affected by an increase in the dose per fraction. This means that giving a patient many small doses (hyperfractionation) will not greatly reduce the rate of tumour-cell kill, but will significantly reduce the risk of late side-effects.

Acceleration

In the past, when considering the doubling time of tumours, it was the doubling of the visible or palpable tumour which was measured, and this commonly ranged from 3 to 9 months. It is now also necessary to consider the rate at which the cells divide. The potential doubling time is that required for the cells to double in number if there is no cell loss. Cells may be lost from the cell cycle because of death (largely due to inadequate nutrition), maturation with loss of ability to reproduce, or by going into a resting phase. Before treatment, such cell loss is an advantage because the tumour will increase in bulk more slowly. When treatment by radiotherapy is initiated and many cells are destroyed it is believed that normal cell loss no longer occurs. When testing for the potential cell doubling time of tumours (T_{pot}) it was discovered that many tumours have the potential to double in cell number in only a few days, even in less than 24 hours. It is, therefore, possible for the tumour to double its cell numbers over a weekend without treatment, or even between treatments on consecutive days. To overcome this, the overall treatment time should be reduced and preferably be continuous.

CONTINUOUS HYPERFRACTIONATED ACCELERATED RADIOTHERAPY (CHART)

Taking into account both of the above processes, reduced doses of 1.5 Gy minimum tumour dose (TD_{min}) per fraction (the mean being 2.0 Gy) are given three times a day for 12 consecutive days (Saunders et al., 1991). In this way, treatment is complete before reaction occurs. To allow for the repair of normal tissues within the treatment volume, a gap is needed between treatments. The half-time repair of sublethal injury in most normal tissue is 1–1.5 hours. An interfraction gap of 6 hours is long enough to allow approximately 90% repair of sublethal injury to occur in normal tissue within the treatment volume.

Patient Management

At the centre for Cancer Treatment, Mount Vernon Hospital, it was decided to treat at 08.00, 14.00 and 20.00 hours daily, beginning on a Monday morning and continuing until the following Friday. This would allow for a 6-hour gap between treatments. The planning process is exactly the same as for conventionally treated patients, with both large and reduced volumes being given in the majority of cases. During the first phase of the pilot study, only 1.4 Gy TD_{min} per fraction was given, with the large volume receiving 42 Gy and the small volume 8.4 Gy. After 16 months, when 38 patients had been treated, the dose was increased to 1.5 Gy per fraction, with 42 Gy given to the large volume and 12 Gy to the reduced volume. Following the unexpected finding of radiation myelitis in the head and neck of patients treated, it was decided to reduce the dose to the large volume cases, which included the spinal cord in some cases, whilst keeping the total dose the same. A minimum tumour dose of 37.5 Gy was given to the large volume, and a TD_{min} of 16 Gy was given to the reduced volume. Further biological experiments have now suggested that there is an unusually long repair time for sublethal injury to the spinal cord.

CHART   259

Patients treated under this scheme remain on the hospital site for the 12 days of their treatment, usually in the hostel where they can look after themselves (Wood, 1988).

Pilot Study

By March 1990, 175 patients in total had been treated with CHART (Saunders et al., 1991). Of these, 99 had tumours at the major head and neck sites and 76 had tumours in the bronchus. All patients entered into the CHART bronchus programme had tumours too large or too advanced to be treated with surgery, the primary treatment of choice. Those entered into the head and neck study had large tumours or small tumours with local nodal disease which is not easily cured with conventional radiotherapy fractionation. However, none had distant metastatic disease and no volumes were considered too large for curative treatment. Where possible, the tumour-cell kinetics were determined using bromodeoxyuridine (BrdUdr) injected intravenously which is taken up by cells in the S phase of the cell cycle (Hall, 1978). A biopsy of the tumour was taken approximately 6 hours later and put through the cell sorter in the laboratory. This device counts the number of cells in the sample and shows the number which contain BrdUdr, i.e. those in the S phase at the time of uptake. The proportion of the tumour cells in the S phase and the duration of the cell cycle can be calculated and, from these, the potential cell doubling time (T_{pot}).

The first cohort of patients treated in January 1986 consisted of two head and neck cases and two bronchus cases. It was uncertain how they would react to the treatment and therefore great care was taken to observe and document all reactions. It transpired that during the 12 treatment days little or no reaction was observed at all. On day 15 or 16 (day 1 being the first Monday of treatment) mucositis was seen in the head and neck cases, and by day 17 or 18 oesophagitis was observed in the bronchus cases. These were treated using aspirin mucilage and alteration of the patients' diet to bland, soft items, or fluids. The patients were kept on the ward for 1 month to ensure that no further problems arose. After 3 months, encouraged by the tolerance to treatment and the tumour response, further groups of patients were treated on a regular basis. All patients were seen weekly for 4–6 weeks, with all reactions being documented and coded. A computer database was set up to ensure that all information was collected in the same manner, and that it could be analysed at a later date.

MANAGEMENT OF CHART IN A BUSY RADIOTHERAPY DEPARTMENT

The CHART regime is a change in culture for many radiographers and, as such, careful management of the timetable is essential (Wood, 1988).

A 09.00–17.00 working day is accepted as the norm in most radiotherapy departments, and even providing an on-call service only requires a few evenings or weekends to be given up per year for each radiographer.

To introduce CHART, the co-operation of radiographers is vital. Therapy radiographers have enjoyed being in the front line of research and have become closely involved with all aspects of the trial. The introduction of CHART has been welcomed by most radiographers in centres where it is used.

Only one of the three daily fractions could be incorporated in the normal 09.00–17.00 working day within a busy radiotherapy centre. To ensure that the treatment times are within acceptable hours for both patients and staff, 08.00, 14.00 and 20.00 h seem most appropriate. The machine used for CHART treatments usually extends the day to include the 08.00 treatment by two members of staff arriving early and leaving at 16.00 h, if possible. This means that only the evening and weekend sessions need staffing. Groups of 3–5 patients are put through the CHART regime, which begins on a Monday morning and is completed at 20.00 h on Friday of the following week. The patients are grouped in such a way so as to ensure that each session is over within 1 hour, in order to avoid interrupting the normal day's work. The evening and weekend sessions can be staffed in many different ways:

1. By a fixed rota dictated by the manager.
2. By two or three staff employed especially to cover out-of-hours work.
3. By volunteers from the existing staff.

The first option has the advantage that all staff have to be involved and that the manager is sure that staff familiar with the patients and the machines are involved. The second option may be useful if local staff are not interested in working out of hours, and the job may suit qualified personnel who find short fixed hours convenient. The third option finds favour with staff in as much as it allows them to earn extra money for the overtime hours worked. Problems arise when staff have arranged to work on a session having never seen the patient set-up. In addition, some method of ensuring that at least one member of the

CHART   261

team is of a senior grade must be in place. Therefore, this option also requires some management control.

Patients going through the CHART regime need to consent to the treatment being given, as do all patients, but in this case an explanation of the research aspects of their management must be included. It is a debatable point as to whether patients who are included in a research project *may* do better as the care they receive is often more personalized and less 'rushed' in appearance. The patient knows he or she is special and this gives many positive benefits.

RESULTS

The results of the pilot study have been published previously (Saunders et al., 1991). Here, only the main benefits seen in these groups of patients are described. Figure 24.2 gives data for fraction doses of both 1.4 and 1.5 Gy TD_{min}. It can be seen that there is significant benefit to both the head and neck and bronchus cases.

In April 1990, the study became a randomized, multicentre trial, and protocols to suit all centres involved were written by the CHART Steering Committee, backed by the Medical Research Council, Cancer Research Campaign and Department of Health. These protocols are extremely prescriptive, trying to ensure that all patients are treated in exactly the same way. Rigorous quality-assurance programmes were also set up to provide proof that the protocols were adhered to.

One major aspect of the pilot study was changed in the randomized trial. It was decided to follow international recommendations and prescribe to the intersection point of the treatment beams, as opposed to the TD_{min}. This had the effect of reducing the dose given to the patient by around 5% (Figure 24.3). This may well be clinically significant and thus the results of the randomized study may not be as predicted by the pilot study (Dische et al., 1993). Certainly, in studies of tumours in mice a reduction of dose by 5% reduced the tumour control probability by 25%. This refers to homogeneous tumours of a very small size not comparable in every way to human tumours, but there is an indication that this dose reduction may indeed cause reduced tumour control.

Entry into the trial has been very satisfactory and will close to new patients in March 1995. With almost 1300 patients entered into the randomized study 1 year before it is closed, a vast databank will be available for analysis.

The CHART study has shown the possibility of an increase in cure rates and a reduction in morbidity, the achievement of either of which

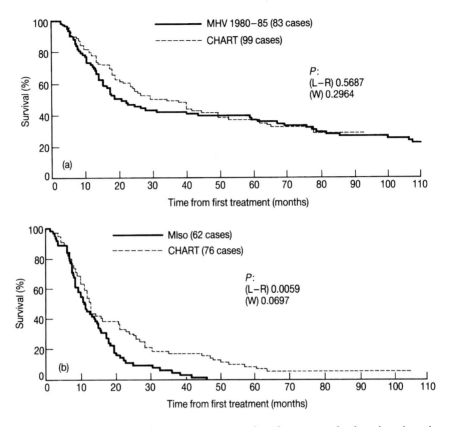

Figure 24.2 (a) Survival in patients treated with CHART for head and neck tumours compared with a conventionally treated and matched group. (b) Survival in patients treated with CHART for bronchus tumours compared with a group previously treated in the misonidazole study with conventional fractionation.

would justify its continued use. Socio-economic studies carried out by the University of York Health Economics Group on patients entered into the CHART trial will also provide key information on how CHART treatment may be arranged in the future.

FUTURE

CHART may be the future for some specific tumours. It may be that the results from the CHART randomized study will point the way to new areas of research. Already accelerated radiotherapy with carbogen and

CHART   263

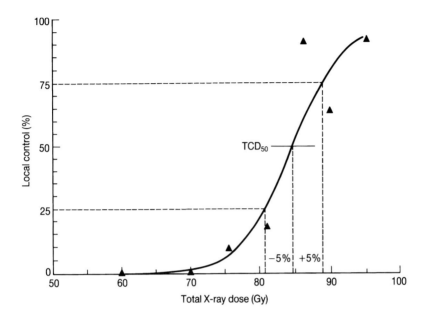

Figure 24.3   Experiments in mice illustrate how a dose reduction of 5% can potentially reduce the tumour control probability by 25% in homogeneous tumours of small size.

nicotinamide (ARCON) (Hoskin and Saunders, 1994) is being studied using CHART as the radiotherapy fractionation standard. CHART plus a high-dose rate (HDR) afterloading for reduced volumes in oesophageal tumours has been looked at in a few cases, and CHARTWEL (CHART weekend less) is being offered to bronchus patients whose tumours are too large for inclusion in the CHART randomized study.

In one form or another, CHART is here to stay.

References

Dische, S., Saunders, M.I., Williams, C. et al. (1993) Precision in reporting the dose given in a course of radiotherapy. *Radiotherapy and Oncology* **29:** 287–293.

Hall, E. (1978) *Radiobiology for the Radiologist.* London: Harper & Row.

Hoskin, P.J., Saunders, M.I. (1994) ARCON. *Clinical Oncology* **6:** 281–282.

Saunders, M.I., Dische, S., Grosch, E.J. et al. (1991) Experience with CHART. *International Journal of Radiation Oncology, Biology, Physics* **21:** 871–878.

Wood, J.M. (1988) The management of accelerated hyperfractionation in radiotherapy. MDCR Thesis, College of Radiographers, London.

25

A Multidisciplinary Approach to Cancer Patients

Judy Young

INTRODUCTION

Cancer represents chaos. Chaos is the lack of central control, the lack of direction, goal and organisation. Chaos is madness within a system. Yet new order grows out of chaos as a natural process. Having cancer creates chaos in the body, mind and the family. Intervention – medical, psychological, social or spiritual – is aimed at trying to regain control and a sense of direction. Direction and control create movement; movement brings hope. (Kfir and Slevin, 1991)

A diagnosis of cancer represents an existential crisis generated by recognition of the basic insecurity of the human condition and of the necessity of facing mortality. Many people receiving a diagnosis of cancer experience a sense of loss of control over both their bodies and their lives in general (Moorey et al., 1989:15). This experience can manifest itself in feelings of helplessness and hopelessness related to the uncertainty of prognosis, together with feelings of inadequacy resulting in an impaired ability to perform everyday tasks (Moorey et al., 1989:15).

Cancer therapies, frequently viewed with such fear and anxiety, may also fuel these feelings of loss of control and add to the sense of helplessness already experienced by some patients. Side-effects of treatment, such as worry about the future, concern for family and friends, changes in appearance and effects on career and status, all serve to increase the feeling of chaos and confusion which surround the diagnosis and treatment of cancer. Hopefully, the patient will emerge out of this chaos and confusion with a newfound direction and better coping skills in order to deal with the crisis. However, in the majority of cases this cannot be achieved in isolation, and the patient needs help from a number of sources to guide him or her through the cancer journey.

By the time a crisis occurs it may be too late to introduce a new supportive framework for the patient. It is important that all professional and lay carers of cancer patients are able to identify and build on existing sources of strength. Because the issues are complex and a wide range of people may be involved with a patient, a 'team approach', involving family, hospital, community and lay support, is essential to address the needs and wishes of the patient and family at each stage of the cancer journey. As helping people with cancer needs more knowledge, skill and time than any one person can offer, these needs are best met by a multidisciplinary team. The members of this team need a working knowledge and understanding of the role of other team members, other professionals and any lay support bodies outside the team. They also need the ability to recognize the most appropriate way to help a patient at a particular time, and indeed when support from another patient or a volunteer may be more appropriate.

THE CANCER JOURNEY

A patient's cancer journey may be just a few months or several years. During this time the patient may only attend the cancer treatment centre for 2 or 3 months, obtaining the majority of care or treatment in the local community.

Along the cancer journey patients will interact with professionals from a range of disciplines, who may or may not meet their needs. At each stage it is important that professionals are totally patient focused, so that patients' actual needs are addressed, rather than what the professional perceives as patients' needs. It is important also to recognize that each patient is an individual, and that to be too prescriptive about their needs is to disregard that individuality.

STAGES OF THE CANCER JOURNEY

Diagnosis

The journey may begin with a range of symptoms which lead to a visit to the general practitioner (GP), where the diagnosis is made and the initial 'bad news' broken. Buckman (1984) states that bad news is any information likely to drastically alter a patient's view of his or her future, including any alteration to expected life-span

Regardless of how the diagnosis is made, whether the cancer is anticipated or is found randomly at screening (for example, on a routine mammogram), the patient will experience initial shock, which requires time, reassurance and information. A patient's perception of whether the cancer will shorten life is particularly important in determining adjustment to the disease. (Moorey et al., 1989:13)

The patient may receive professional support at this stage from the GP, surgeon, or a specialist support nurse such as a breast care nurse. The GP is the focal point for results of tests, scans and X-rays, and probably the one constant factor during the cancer journey, so it is vital for a patient to develop a good relationship with him or her. Specialist nurses, often working closely with surgeons, offer support, information, education, advice and counselling to patients and their families. They are generally hospital based and, where appropriate, can help with decisions about treatment options. Patients' choices are strongly influenced by what they perceive their doctors want them to do, and a doctor's recommendations are often subject to bias (Penman et al., 1984). Removing bias from the presentation of choice can be difficult. The role of the specialist nurse is to discuss the options with the patient and to help him or her make treatment decisions with as little professional bias as possible.

A patient may also need access to people who have had similar cancers and who have survived. There are a number of self-help and support organizations (Table 25.1) available which offer an opportunity for people with cancer and their relatives and friends to share feelings and gain support and encouragement from each other. Based on the principle of self-help they complement rather than replace professional care.

Table 25.1 National support organizations

BACUP 3 Bath Place, Rivington Street, London EC2A 3JR (Tel. 0171-613 2121)
Cancerlink 17 Britannia Street, London WC1X 9JN (Tel. 0171-833 3451)
Hodgkin's Disease Association P.O. Box 275, Haddenham, Aylesbury, Bucks HP17 8JJ (Tel. 01844 291500)
Leukaemia Care Society 14 Kingfisher Court, Verney Bridge, Pinhoe, Exeter, Devon EX4 8JN (Tel. 01392 64848)

Treatment

The options for treating cancer are radiotherapy, chemotherapy, surgery, or a combination of all three. The patient should be invited to attend hospital appointments with a relative or close friend who can provide moral or practical support. If the patient wishes, it can be helpful for the relative or friend to be present at the consultation with the doctor. This can help the patient to assimilate information about the disease and make useful decisions about its management.

Surgery

During the hospital stay the patient may interact with surgeons, anaesthetists, specialist nurses, (for example, stoma care nurses), surgical-appliance officers, ward nurses, dietitians, occupational therapists, physiotherapists, counsellors, social workers, clergy, house officers, registrars, consultants and diagnostic radiographers. The patient may be confused about the roles of this mass of people and how they interact. It is vital that each member of the team is aware of the needs of an individual patient, otherwise there may be an assumption that someone else has addressed them.

Meetings between the different health-care professionals involved in the care of a cancer patient provide an opportunity and focus for the exchange of information and the formulation of an integrated approach to care. On discharge from hospital, aftercare plans and appointments should be organized with the patient, family and relevant professionals. Communications from hospital to GPs, district nurses and Macmillan nurses, for example, are a crucial part of any discharge plan.

Radiotherapy

The patient may interact with physicists, radiographers, student radiographers, mould-room technicians, oncologists, clinic nurses, counsellors, dietitians and physiotherapists during radiotherapy. This again may be very confusing for the patient, and all professional staff should be aware of the issues important to each patient, and ready to address any problems.

Although radiotherapy is one of the most effective treatments for cancer, the time actually spent by each patient in a radiotherapy department is minimal compared with the time spent back in the community. Nevertheless, radiographers build up intense and highly supportive relationships with patients over a short period of time, and can influence considerably not only how the patient is treated but also how they may cope with the disease.

The patient will probably interact with radiographers more than any other professional group during radiotherapy. The same team of radiographers may treat a patient daily for up to 6 weeks, providing a tremendous potential to build up a good rapport but on a busy linear accelerator 40–50 patients may be treated in a day, so it is difficult to provide full support to each patient. Nevertheless, the radiographer seeing a patient daily is ideally placed to recognize signs and symptoms of distress, pick up cues, and ask focused questions to make a quick assessment of his or her concerns. It is important that the radiographer then refers the patient to the most appropriate person to deal with the problem.

During treatment many patients suffer from physical and emotional side-effects, such as skin reactions and depression. It is important that patients are listened to, reassured, supported and offered sound practical advice to help them cope.

The patient may not feel better for weeks or even months after treatment has finished. Supportive care should be offered and organized, if required, at the end of treatment. Many patients find a comforting link in telephone helplines, which are offered by some hospitals and national support organizations such as BACUP (British Association of Cancer United Patients) or the Hodgkin's Disease Association.

At the end of radiotherapy patients often have a sense of anti-climax in addition to feeling unwell, tired and depressed. Despite undergoing intensive treatment many feel worse rather than better and are unable to distinguish between symptoms of the disease and side-effects of treatment. They are also living with the chronic uncertainty of not knowing whether their cancer has been cured, and may find this feeling very difficult to live with.

Some people may benefit from sharing these feelings and experiences with other patients at this stage, whilst others may seek reassurance from their GP, Macmillan nurse or oncologist. Radiographers can play a major role, before the treatment finishes, by warning patients and their families of the possibility, and normality, of such feelings.

Chemotherapy

During chemotherapy the patient will interact with chemotherapy nurses, doctors and other patients. Patients can gain a tremendous amount of support and encouragement from each other whilst undergoing chemotherapy. Shared experiences of dealing with nausea and hair loss can provide a significant degree of support (and stress!) amongst patients sitting together in waiting rooms, or on wards.

A small number of patients develop anticipatory nausea and vomiting as a conditioned response to chemotherapy. They may be desensitized to these effects by using cognitive/behavioural techniques such as relaxation and visualization, which may require appointments with counsellors or psychologists. Burish et al. (1987) showed that patients were able to reduce the severity of nausea and vomiting both during and after chemotherapy by using such techniques.

The major problems experienced by patients undergoing chemotherapy are nausea and altered body image, such as hair loss and weight gain (with steroids). Distress is also caused by loss of fertility and libido; these problems are not easily dealt with and require a sensitive team approach using the appropriate professional or non-professional discipline.

A small number of patients develop clinical anxiety or depression whilst undergoing cancer treatments; they may require psychotropic medication in the form of antidepressant or anxiolytic drugs. Whilst some oncologists and GPs are happy to prescribe these drugs, others prefer to refer the patient for a psychiatric assessment.

Because of the stigma attached to such intervention, many patients are reluctant or indeed refuse to be referred to a psychiatrist and may suffer needlessly. Where a liaison psychiatrist is part of the cancer support team, the patient may feel less stigmatized by seeing just 'another' member of the team for help with their problems.

Follow-up and Ongoing Care

Once treatment has finished, the patient can often feel very isolated unless a good support system has been identified. Many have difficulty because, without a definite pronouncement of 'cure' from their doctor, follow-up appointments are awaited both with hope and dread – hope that the doctor can provide reassurance that the cancer has definitely gone, and dread that it might have returned. The majority of patients do not understand why they are not scanned at each follow-up appointment, and equally are unsure when or whether to report symptoms such as aches and pains.

The experience of a life-threatening disease such as cancer makes people feel vulnerable and frightened. This may give them an over-anxious preoccupation with their body so that a 'normal' ache or pain takes on massive and sinister proportions, leading to chronic fear and anxiety.

The patient's family can help greatly at this stage by offering support, reassurance and distractions. It is clear that the ongoing supportive care of the cancer patient cannot remain in the domain of the professionals, other than to provide medical advice and reassurance related to symptoms and possible long-term side-effects of treatment.

The needs of a particular patient and family will differ according to the phase of the illness, and different phases and forms of cancer may present different issues for patient and family care and support (Bluglass, 1986). Some find support groups for patients and/or relatives helpful at this time, whilst others may want to share their feelings and uncertainties with counsellors with a knowledge of cancer.

The needs of patients' children may be overlooked, and require keen observation and attention. When one member of a family becomes ill the needs of the rest of the family may be ignored, whilst attention is focused on the sick person. Children often exhibit attention-seeking behaviour, which may result in punishment rather than understanding if not recognized as such. Occasionally children may require professional help and, through the GP, it may be possible to arrange either for a child psychologist to visit the home or for the child to attend a clinic. If the psychologist is identified as part of the team then the parents will be less likely to feel stigmatized by such intervention.

Relapse, Recurrence and Palliative Treatment

The stage of the journey when relapse or recurrence is diagnosed is often more traumatic for the patient than the original diagnosis. The fear and dread which has haunted them for months or years has finally materialized – the disease has returned and the reality of the situation begins to dawn. The treatment offered at this stage depends on the type and site of cancer, ranging from further intensive chemotherapy (for example, relapse of Hodgkin's disease) to palliative radiotherapy for widespread bony metastases. The patient will interact with similar health-care professionals to those met in the early treatment stages, but more supportive and emotional interventions will be required.

Radiographers involved in treating recurrent cancer will be aware that radiation doses are much lower and given over shorter periods of time, and that less complicated and time-consuming techniques will be employed. The emphasis now is very much on symptom control and improving quality of life, and patient comfort should become of paramount importance.

When treating patients with palliative radiotherapy it is important that radiographers recognize the context in which the treatment is undertaken and that where possible treatment is organized in conjunction with other supportive modalities, particularly for inpatients. Outpatients may find greater difficulty in travelling to and from the hospital and need to rely heavily on family, friends or volunteers for transport.

Patients with recurrent disease may be visited regularly at home by a Macmillan nurse, who will help to organize symptom control and drugs, as well as talking to the patient in the context of the family and helping them to adjust to the new situation.

Stam et al. (1986) drew attention to the fact that cancer patients' concern about the effect of their illness on the family is greater than their own concern about the illness itself. This needs sensitive handling, as both patient and family may be trying to protect one another from the pain of realizing the seriousness of the situation.

Frequently, relatives will wish to accompany patients on visits to radiotherapy and to be with the patient for as much of the time as possible. This should be taken into account when providing adequate waiting space for sick patients. Quiet rooms for relatives should also be made available for more private conversations with staff when necessary.

The Terminal Phase

The terminal phase of the cancer journey often begins with the realization that death is going to happen within the near future. Loss of physical and mental control frequently occurs and patients and relatives find difficulty in adjusting to the reality of the situation.

Not all communication within the cancer care field is with patients or their families, as working in the field of terminal disease means working with a wide variety of different professionals, volunteers and public or charitable organizations whose services or interventions are needed.

With cure no longer an option, specialists in the field of terminal care are forced to explore new ways of caring. This exploration may uncover the painful gap between the needs of patients and the way in which those needs are being met in hospital and the community (Cassidy, 1991).

Radiotherapy and chemotherapy have little to offer in terminal care, but those involved in treatment of cancer patients have much to learn from the hospice movement in terms of team approach. A successful team approach is based on the recognition that the patient is an individual in their own right and exists on a number of levels: mind, body and spirit.

Dunlop (1993) states that the patient is far more than just a physical illness, and that both the person and their family must be considered the unit of care. The hospice considers the person as a highly individual, complex, interwoven pattern of physical, psychological, social and spiritual dimensions.

An incurable illness such as cancer affects not only the patient, but also family and friends, both whilst the patient is still alive and after death. To address the wide-ranging and complex issues of the dying patient, hospices have available a multidisciplinary team which includes the whole range of health-care professionals as well as volunteer counsellors, priests, rabbis, and other individuals to work with patient and family.

SUMMARY

The aim of an ideal cancer-care service should be to provide an integrated holistic approach which offers a seamless service from diagnosis to death. If it is accepted that an individual exists on several levels (mind, body and spirit), then a truly holistic approach to each patient must be adopted. The most appropriate care should therefore be made available to treat the whole person in the context of their own individual life:

> *The cure of the part should not be attempted without treatment of the whole. No attempt should be made to cure the body without the soul, and thus if the head and body are to be healthy you must begin by curing the mind. That is the first thing. Let no one persuade you to cure the head until he has first given you his soul to be cured. For this is the great error of our day, that physicians first separate the soul from the body. (Plato, 400 BC)*

References

Buckman, R. (1984) Breaking bad news: why is it still so difficult? *British Medical Journal* **288**: 1597-1599.

Bluglass, K. (1986) Caring for the family. In Stoll, B.A. (ed.) *Coping With Cancer Stress* Lancaster: Nijhoff.

Burish, T.G., Carey, M.P., Krozely, M.G. (1987) Conditioned side-effects induced by cancer chemotherapy; prevention through behavioural treatment. *Journal of Consulting and Clinical Psychology* **55:** 42-48.

Cassidy, S. (1991) Terminal care. In Watson, M. (ed.) *Cancer Patient Care.* Cambridge: Cambridge University Press.

Dunlop, R. (1993) Wider applications of palliative care. In Saunders, C. (ed.) *The Management of Terminal Malignant Disease* London: Hodder & Stoughton.

Kfir, N., Slevin, M. (1991) *Challenging Cancer: From Chaos to Control.* London: Tavistock/Routledge.

Moorey, S., Greer, S. (1989) *Psychological Therapy for Patients with Cancer.* Oxford: Heinemann Medical.

Penman, D.T., Holland, J.C., Bahma, G.F. (1984) Informed consent for investigational chemotherapy: patients' and physicians' perceptions. *Journal of Clinical Oncology* **2:** 849-855.

Stam, H.J., Bultz, B.D., Pittman, C.A. (1986) Psychosocial problems and interventions in a referred sample of cancer patients. *Psychosomatic Medicine* **48:** 539-548.

26

Imaging Services in the Community

Alexander J. M. Cavenagh

BACKGROUND

The philosophy which denied general practitioners (GPs) access to most radiology services in the mistaken belief that this would economize its use has vanished but mammography is still subject to this jurassic embargo in the hope that co-ordinated breast cancer services will arise. These may be some time in coming. The managerial pendulum has now swung with a vengeance to a state where providers and trusts, in their search for business, are competing to bring services to the community. All of this is good news for patients, and primary care generally. Gone, too, are the days when the activities of radiologists were limited by plain and contrast X-rays, where their clinical input was limited to the reading of films and writing of reports in what, all too frequently, were inadequate and poorly lighted offices. Competition and incentives are likely to produce profound and rapid changes in community imaging services, driven by GP fundholders on the one hand and the more entrepreneurial National Health Service (NHS) trusts on the other.

Explosion of Services

The advent of ultrasound, computed tomography (CT) scanning and magnetic resonance imaging (MRI) has combined to make the radiology department the absolute lynchpin of diagnosis, and in many cases of therapy, in much of Western medicine. Specialism within departments now means that for a district general hospital (DGH) at least four consultant radiologists must be appointed. They will have special interests in ultrasound, CT, MRI, interventional procedures such as angioplasty, isotope investigations and the traditional bread-and-butter plain X-ray and contrast media examinations which have been the bedrock of the service since Röntgen himself. Each specialism develops a team of expert radiographers, technicians and secretariat. Ideally, these will extend their tentacles to provide cover and advice for surrounding community hospitals and general practices, rooting the service solidly to the population served. Debate now centres on where expensive facilities can most logically be centred and the extent to which the majority of low-technology services can safely and economically be moved to the periphery.

In the majority of community hospitals, building and revenue costs run at approximately 65% of those of DGHs (Netton, 1994; Tucker and Bosanquet, unpublished). Average unit costs of a particular service per user will be affected by the level of spare capacity. If imaging facilities and staff are underused when located in community hospitals, unit costs may rise. But this would need to be set against the additional quality advantages to patients of receiving services near to their homes and the consequent savings in time and loss of work for patients. When ambulance and other travelling costs are taken into account, a calculation so far unpublished, the reasons for providing the maximum amount of imaging services in the community are compelling. Amazingly, at a time of considerable community hospital development in most areas, there are still threats of closure in others. Published authoritative studies of costings will be essential to decide this issue. However, it is a mistake to consider imaging services in isolation.

A serious effort to cash in on the cost benefits of community, rather than central, provision will mean that the majority of hospital services which do not require high-tech DGH or regional hospital care must be provided locally also. Community hospital care will become the norm rather than the exception and the resulting savings can be devoted to service improvements at all levels. At present, the size, scope and variety of community hospitals is such that in some instances the community hospital provides all services to a level which appears almost to compete with those of the DGH. At the other end of the scale a considerable number of community hospitals are doing little more, in clinical terms, than the provision of excellent nursing-home facilities. Efforts to prescribe norms and to standardize arrangements appear to be misguided. The history, staffing and traditions of each hospital are as unique as the community it serves, and new hospitals will inevitably be slotted into an existing framework of care which has run for many years. However, it appears correct to stretch the frontiers of what can be provided locally insofar as is possible. Hence, community hospitals should perform the majority of procedures which, in the DGH, would fall to staff of subconsultant grade and should be equipped to provide this level of service.

Costs

At 1994 prices, the approximate costs of equipping a simple department for diagnostic x-ray services is £60 000 with an expected life of apparatus of 10–15 years. Simple, state-of-the-art ultrasound apparatus adds £30 000. The revenue costs of staffing must include an adequate rota of radiographers, including an experienced ultrasound operator and consultant sessions to cover supervision of the department, reading of films and screening of contrast-media examinations if these are to be offered. An immediate resuscitation service must also be available if contrast-media examinations are to be available. The impact of daylight processing and laser imager systems for departments whose workloads justify the expense will be to produce a more rapid and better reported service.

REQUIREMENTS AND EQUIPMENT

X-rays

The immediate need for any community is for a casualty service. In terms of efficiency to the local population this is the most effective service that community hospitals provide, with an onward referral rate of only 2% (Cavenagh, 1978). Much of the work that comes into casualty departments, wherever they are located, is simply primary care by other means and well within the competence of nurse practitioners and GPs. An x-ray service to provide extremity and chest films within normal working hours is the minimal imaging requirement to support a community hospital casualty service. The value of contrast-media examinations will remain for investigations of renal colic and haema-

Index